T0259334

Low Back Pain

Guest Editor

ERON G. MANUSOV, MD

PRIMARY CARE:
CLINICS IN OFFICE PRACTICE

www.primarycare.theclinics.com

Consulting Editor
JOEL J. HEIDELBAUGH, MD

September 2012 • Volume 39 • Number 3

SAUNDERS an imprint of ELSEVIER, Inc.

W.B. SAUNDERS COMPANY
A Division of Elsevier Inc.

1600 John F. Kennedy Boulevard, Suite 1800 • Philadelphia, PA 19103-2899

http://www.theclinics.com

PRIMARY CARE: CLINICS IN OFFICE PRACTICE Volume 39, Number 3
September 2012 ISSN 0095-4543, ISBN-13: 978-1-4557-4936-2

Editor: Yonah Korngold

© **2012 Elsevier Inc. All rights reserved.**

This journal and the individual contributions contained in it are protected under copyright by Elsevier, and the following terms and conditions apply to their use:

Photocopying
Single photocopies of single articles may be made for personal use as allowed by national copyright laws. Permission of the Publisher and payment of a fee is required for all other photocopying, including multiple or systematic copying, copying for advertising or promotional purposes, resale, and all forms of document delivery. Special rates are available for educational institutions that wish to make photocopies for non-profit educational classroom use. For information on how to seek permission visit www.elsevier.com/permissions or call: (+44) 1865 843830 (UK)/(+1) 215 239 3804 (USA).

Derivative Works
Subscribers may reproduce tables of contents or prepare lists of articles including abstracts for internal circulation within their institutions. Permission of the Publisher is required for resale or distribution outside the institution. Permission of the Publisher is required for all other derivative works, including compilations and translations (please consult www.elsevier.com/permissions).

Electronic Storage or Usage
Permission of the Publisher is required to store or use electronically any material contained in this journal, including any article or part of an article (please consult www.elsevier.com/permissions). Except as outlined above, no part of this publication may be reproduced, stored in a retrieval system or transmitted in any form or by any means, electronic, mechanical, photocopying, recording or otherwise, without prior written permission of the Publisher.

Notice
No responsibility is assumed by the Publisher for any injury and/or damage to persons or property as a matter of products liability, negligence or otherwise, or from any use or operation of any methods, products, instructions or ideas contained in the material herein. Because of rapid advances in the medical sciences, in particular, independent verification of diagnoses and drug dosages should be made.

Although all advertising material is expected to conform to ethical (medical) standards, inclusion in this publication does not constitute a guarantee or endorsement of the quality or value of such product or of the claims made of it by its manufacturer.

Primary Care: Clinics in Office Practice (ISSN: 0095–4543) is published quarterly by Elsevier Inc., 360 Park Avenue South, New York, NY 10010-1710. Months of issue are March, June, September, and December. Periodicals postage paid at New York, NY and additional mailing offices. Subscription prices are $216.00 per year (US individuals), $353.00 (US institutions), $108.00 (US students), $264.00 (Canadian individuals), $415.00 (Canadian institutions), $169.00 (Canadian students), $329.00 (international individuals), $415.00 (international institutions), and $169.00 (international students). Foreign air speed delivery is included in all *Clinics* subscription prices. All prices are subject to change without notice. POSTMASTER: Send address changes to *Primary Care: Clinics in Office Practice*, Elsevier Periodicals Customer Service, 11830 Westline Industrial Drive, St. Louis, MO 63146. Customer Service Health Sciences Division, Subscription Customer Service, 3251 Riverport Lane, Maryland Heights, MO 63043. **Customer Service: 1-800-654-2452 (U.S. and Canada); 314-447-8871 (outside U.S. and Canada). Fax: 314-447-8029. E-mail: journalscustomerservice-usa@elsevier.com (for print support); journalsonlinesupport-usa@elsevier.com (for online support).**

Reprints. For copies of 100 or more, of articles in this publication, please contact the Commercial Reprints Department, Elsevier Inc., 360 Park Avenue South, New York, NY 10010-1710. Tel. (212) 633-3812; Fax: (212) 482-1935; E-mail: reprints@elsevier.com.

Primary Care: Clinics in Office Practice is covered in *MEDLINE/PubMed (Index Medicus)* and *EMBASE/ Excerpta Medica, Current Contents/Clinical Medicine,* and *ISI/BIOMED.*

Printed and bound by CPI Group (UK) Ltd, Croydon, CR0 4YY

Transferred to Digital Print 2012

Contributors

CONSULTING EDITOR

JOEL J. HEIDELBAUGH, MD, FAAFP, FACG
Clinical Assistant Professor and Clerkship Director, Department of Family Medicine; Clinical Assistant Professor, Department of Urology, University of Michigan Medical School, Ann Arbor, Michigan

GUEST EDITOR

ERON G. MANUSOV, MD
Vice President, Clinical and Educational Services; Program Director, Family Medicine Residency, Duke Southern Regional AHEC, Fayetteville, North Carolina

AUTHORS

ERIC L. GARLAND, PhD
Assistant Professor, College of Social Work, Trinity Institute for the Addictions, Florida State University, Tallahassee, Florida

BIKRAMJIT S. GREWAL, MD
Orthopedic Surgery Resident (PGY-5), University of Chapel Hill, North Carolina

HARKIRAN GREWAL, MD
Southern Regional AHEC, Fayetteville, North Carolina

DONALD GRANT GUILD, MD
Southern Regional AHEC, Fayetteville, North Carolina

DONALD C. MAHARTY, DO
Associate Professor in Family Medicine; Director of Medical Education for the VCOM/DUKE-Southern Regional AHEC Family Medicine Residency, Southern Regional AHEC, Fayetteville, North Carolina

ERON G. MANUSOV, MD
Vice President, Clinical and Educational Services; Program Director, Family Medicine Residency, Duke Southern Regional AHEC, Fayetteville, North Carolina

DAN MARLOWE, PhD, LMFT
Department of Applied Psychosocial Medicine, Southern Regional Area Health Education Center, Fayetteville, North Carolina

SUSAN M. MILLER, PharmD, MBA, BCPS, FCCP
Director of Pharmacotherapy Education, Duke/Southern Regional Area Health Education Family Medicine Residency Program; Clinical Associate Professor, Eshelman School of Pharmacy, University of North Carolina Chapel Hill; Pharmacy Residency Program Director, Cape Fear Valley/Southern Regional Area Health Education Center, Fayetteville, North Carolina

SHARI ELIZABETH NOKES
Esq., Nokes & Nokes, A Law Corporation, Aliso Viejo, California

BEAU JAMES NOKES
Esq., Nokes & Nokes, A Law Corporation, Aliso Viejo, California

RASHITA PATEL, MD
Southern Regional AHEC, Fayetteville, North Carolina

STEPHEN QUINTERO, MD
Assistant Professor, College of Medicine, Florida State University, Tallahassee, Florida

JOSÉ E. RODRÍGUEZ, MD
Associate Professor, Department of Family Medicine and Rural Health, The Florida State University College of Medicine, Tallahassee, Florida

LENNY SALZBERG, MD
Associate Director, Family Medicine Residency; Director, Faculty Development Fellowship, Duke/Southern Regional AHEC, Fayetteville, North Carolina

REBEKAH SPROUSE, MD
Southern Regional AHEC, Fayetteville, North Carolina

Contents

treated in the primary care environment, provided the physician has enough knowledge of the medications used to treat low back pain. The main treatment goal for acute low back pain is to control the pain and maintain function. For patients with chronic back pain, the goal is continual pain management and prevention of future exacerbations. This article reviews current pharmacological options for the treatment of low back pain, and possible future innovations.

Physical therapy and manual medicine for low back pain encompass many different treatment modalities. There is a vast variety of techniques that physical therapists commonly use in the treatment of low back pain. Some of the therapies include, but are certainly not limited to, education, exercise, lumbar traction, manual manipulation, application of heat, cryotherapy, and ultrasonography. Many of these approaches are discussed specifically in this article.

A variety of nonoperative interventions are available to treat back pain. Careful assessment, discussion, and planning need to be performed to individualize care to each patient. This article discusses good to fair evidence from randomized controlled trials that injection therapy, percutaneous intradiscal radiofrequency thermocoagulation, intradiscal electrothermal therapy, and prolotherapy are not effective. Evidence is poor from randomized controlled trials regarding local injections, Botox, and coblation nucleoplasty; however, with a focused approach, the right treatment can be provided for the right patient. To be more effective in management of back pain, further high-grade randomized controlled trials on efficacy and safety are needed.

There is a need for quality trials that study optimal selection and timing of surgical treatment options. Studies are needed of cost-effectiveness and effect on long-term improvement. Until data from such studies are available, primary physicians should follow the guidelines on conservative management and aggressively evaluate the red flags of low back pain, immediately refer for neurologic deficit and bowel or bladder compromise, and focus treatment on modalities with high-quality evidence-based information. Patients who do not improve can be referred to surgeons with experience and expertise in discectomies.

Complementary and alternative medicine, often referred to as integrated medicine, is often used for the treatment of low back pain. This article presents 6 therapies (ie, behavioral treatment, acupuncture, manipulation, prolotherapy, neuroreflexotherapy, and herbal treatments), which are discussed in terms of the specifics of the modality, as well as the empirical evidence related to their effectiveness.

PRIMARY CARE:
CLINICS IN OFFICE PRACTICE

FORTHCOMING ISSUE

December 2012
Practice Management
Michelle Bholat, MD, *Guest Editor*

RECENT ISSUES

June 2012
Chronic Disease Management
Brooke Salzman, MD,
Lauren Collins, MD, and
Emily R. Hajjar, PharmD, *Guest Editors*

March 2012
Prenatal Care
David R. Harnisch Sr, MD,
Guest Editor

December 2011
Immunizations
Marc Altshuler, MD, and
Edward Buchanan, MD,
Guest Editors

DOWNLOAD
Free App!

Review Articles
THE CLINICS

NOW AVAILABLE FOR YOUR iPhone and iPad

Foreword

"A Pain in the Back"

Acute and chronic low back pain remain among the most common reasons that patients present in primary care. 47.5 million US adults (21.8%) reported a disability in 2005 with Back or Spine problems as the second leading cause.[1] A household interview of a sample of civilian, noninstitutionalized US adults derived from the National Health Interview Survey asked "During the past three months, did you have low back pain?" Respondents were instructed to report pain that had lasted a whole day or more, and conversely, not to report fleeting or minor aches or pains. The survey found that women were more likely than men to have experienced low back pain (30.2% vs 26.0%) within the last month.[2]

What goes through our minds when we see a patient with a chief complaint of low back pain on our schedule? Opportunity toward improvement or despair of chronicity? Frustration due to the impending request for narcotics or completion of disability forms? Optimism of reassurance that over 90% of patients with low back pain are symptom-free within 4 weeks? As complicated as acute and chronic low back pain are, it always seems that an accurate diagnosis remains a challenge through a detailed clinical examination, and prospects for treatment range from physical to pharmacotherapy, various interventional techniques aimed at decreasing pain and improving mobility and function, and surgical decompression and stabilization.

Primary care clinicians often feel that they lack the skills, time, and resources to adequately treat their patients' low back pain. Dr Manusov and his colleagues have done an exceptional job of creating a comprehensive and unique volume of articles dedicated to the challenges of diagnosis and management of low back pain. Impressively, this volume walks the clinician through a detailed discussion of the pathophysiology of the muscular and nervous systems, followed by several articles highlighting various diagnostic and therapeutic modalities. Ever important to the primary care clinician, the articles that are presented outline alternative therapies, as well as the disability examination and inherent medical-legal issues. It is our collective aspiration that this volume will enhance the care of patients with low back pain whom we treat, make the process of caring for them easier, and not have us view the prospect of lumbago simply as a "pain in the back."

Joel J. Heidelbaugh, MD, FAAFP, FACG
Departments of Family Medicine and Urology
University of Michigan Medical School
Ann Arbor, MI 48109, USA

Ypsilanti Health Center
200 Arnet Street, Suite 200
Ypsilanti, MI 48198, USA

E-mail address:
jheidel@umich.edu

Prim Care Clin Office Pract 39 (2012) ix–x
http://dx.doi.org/10.1016/j.pop.2012.06.015
primarycare.theclinics.com
0095-4543/12/$ – see front matter © 2012 Elsevier Inc. All rights reserved.

REFERENCES

1. Brault M. Americans with disabilities: 2005, current population reports, P70-117, Washington, DC: US Census Bureau; 2008. Available at: http://www.cdc.gov/Features/dsAdultDisabilityCauses/.
2. Pleis JR, Ward BW, Lucas JW. Summary health statistics for U.S. adults: National Health Interview Survey, 2009 (provisional report). Vital Health Stat 2010;10(249): 1–207. Available at: http://www.cdc.gov/nchs/data/series/sr_10/sr10_249.pdf.

Preface

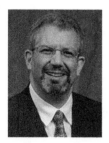

Eron G. Manusov, MD
Guest Editor

The treatment of patients with low back pain, for some primary care physicians, can be a clinical "nightmare." The fact is that we have yet to dramatically improve the diagnosis and treatment of low back pain despite the number of patients with this common ailment. We can blame it primarily on the immensely complicated human skeleton. Starting with the foot and the complicated subtalar joint, forces move up multiple articulations that respond to motion from 360 degrees that transmit energy through and around tendon, muscle, and bone. All these forces result in bone remodeling from pisoelectric forces, changes in tendon strengths, hypertrophy of muscles, growth and death of nerves, and then end up with an eight-pound bowling ball perched on a ring, aptly named the atlas. This chain, called the "back," is positioned and designed to manage an amazingly complex physical existence. Injury to the back and more commonly the low back, however, is common. Amazingly so, the majority of injury to the low back will heal no matter what physicians do. Despite that reassuring truth, it is the remaining large number of patients that present to primary care physicians that we do not know how to appropriately diagnose and treat. A complex musculoskeletal and nervous system complicated by diverse biopsychosocial and cultural differences results in extraordinary diagnostic and treatment dilemmas.

The purpose of the following articles is to review the history of low back pain diagnosis and treatment, present current information on neurocognitive information, and offer systematic evidence-based recommendations for diagnostic and treatment options. Although technology has advanced dramatically during this century, patient outcomes have not followed the same trajectory. Primary care physicians can feel comfortable that information provided and assembled by the authors in the following articles can be a valuable resource to manage patients with low back pain for at least the near future. Hopefully, breakthroughs in medical genetics, physics, chemistry, and neurocognition will necessitate rewriting of the following articles, but until then we hope this edition

Prim Care Clin Office Pract 39 (2012) xi–xii
http://dx.doi.org/10.1016/j.pop.2012.06.001
0095-4543/12/$ – see front matter © 2012 Elsevier Inc. All rights reserved.

primarycare.theclinics.com

will help primary care physicians provide strong evidence-based recommendations to alleviate pain and reduce disability.

Eron G. Manusov, MD
Family Medicine Residency
Duke Southern Regional Area Health Education Center
1601 Owens Drive
Fayetteville, NC 28304, USA

E-mail address:
Eron.Manusov@sr-ahec.org

The History of Lower Back Pain
A Look "Back" Through the Centuries

Donald C. Maharty, DO

KEYWORDS

• Lower back pain • History • Diagnosis • Treatment

KEY POINTS

- The diagnosis and treatment of low back pain must be standardized, based on evidence and solid research.
- The cost to both individuals and society is great and only those diagnostic tests or treatments that can improve the quality and cost of care be advocated.

Throughout history, lower back pain (LBP) has been one of the most common, frustrating, and diagnostically elusive medical maladies of humankind. It frequently reminds us of its presence because it sits in the top 10 list of diagnoses accounting for visits to a primary care office each year.[1] Seventy percent to 85% of patients who seek medical care are affected in their lifetime, costing society billions of dollars annually.[2,3] LBP is challenging for both the patient and the health care provider. On a historical timeline of LBP, we find the earliest surviving documentation originating through Egyptian, Greek, Roman, and Arabic texts. One of the most well-known texts that describes acute lower back strain, the Edwin Smith papyrus **Fig. 1**, dates back to 1500 BC.[4] The following are excerpts from this ancient SOAP note:

1. Examination:

   If thou examinest a man having a sprain of his vertebrae of his spinal column, though shouldst say to him; extend now your legs and contract them both. He contracts them both immediately because of the pain he causes in the vertebrae of the spinal column in which he suffers.

2. Diagnosis:

   Thou shouldst say to him; "On having a sprain in the vertebrae of his spinal column an ailment of which I shall treat."

VCOM/DUKE-Southern Regional AHEC Family Medicine Residency, Southern Regional AHEC, 1601 Owen Drive, Fayetteville, NC 28304, USA
E-mail address: dmmaharty@yahoo.com

Prim Care Clin Office Pract 39 (2012) 463–470
http://dx.doi.org/10.1016/j.pop.2012.06.002
0095-4543/12/$ – see front matter © 2012 Elsevier Inc. All rights reserved.
primarycare.theclinics.com

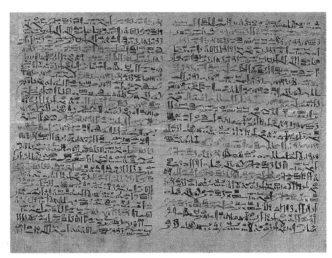

Fig. 1. Plates 6 and 7 of the Edwin Smith Papyrus, the world's oldest surviving surgical document. (*Courtesy of* Rare Book Room, New York Academy of Medicine, New York, NY.)

3. Treatment:

Though shouldst place him prostate on his back.[4]

How far have we come in 3000 years in the accuracy of our diagnosis and treatment of this prevalent ailment? As we travel forward through history, many of the practices of Western medicine can be traced to the *Corpus Hippocraticus* (circa 400 BC), the collected writings of the Greek Library at Cos and Cnidus. It was there that Galen of Pergamon and his disciples dominated the writings for the next 1200 years.[4] Terms such as sciatic pain and LBP were first mentioned by Hippocrates and later Galen, who described back pain in more detail.[5] Most physicians followed Hippocrates' teachings for most of the early centuries of the first millennium. Arabian influence then permeated into the medical landscape with the writing of *The Canons of Medicine* by Avicenna (981–1037).[6] Physicians of the time recommended that surgery could not be performed on the back and most recommendations centered around watchful waiting.

As with many things during medieval times, medical thought, or at least documentation of thought, almost ceased to progress during the Dark Ages, as patient care moved into the hands of the church-state authority. Priests were trained in medicine but care was highly compromised by religious doctrine. Back pain persisted in folk medicine.[4] The Welsh name "shot of the elf" and the Germanic "witch's shot" reflect the belief that pain was caused by external and spiritual influences.[7]

It was only during the twentieth century that physicians seemed to start questioning the certainty of their specific diagnostic acumen of LBP. At the beginning of the century, the cause of LBP was simplified and blamed on either neuritis/neuralgia or muscle rheumatism.[4,6] In the 1920s and 1930s, theories grew and coexisted. Neurasthenia, hysteria, nervousness, neurosis, psychogenesis, and psychosomatic origin were terms to describe psychogenic causes for LBP.[4] During the Second World War, hysterical sciatica and lumbago occurred more often than during peaceful times.[7,8] The use of the descriptive identifying disk disease was not even mentioned in studies as a specific disease entity until the latter half of the twentieth century. Then in the 1940s, the dynasty of the disk paradigm dominated almost all discussion.[9,10] This topic faded as further investigation revealed disk disease accounting for only less than 10% to 15% of LBP.[4,9,10] As technology advanced, physicians tended to trust the results of their diagnostic instruments more than the physical examination, even despite knowing that bulging or herniated disks and symptom production have a poor correlation.[11,12] Later studies describe an 80% uncertainty about the specific cause of LBP, and medical science began to question, "Is there any progress in our understanding?"[13–15] The terminology of mechanical LBP dominates the generally accepted etiologic description for the complicated differential diagnosis of LBP because this term encompasses 97% of the possible diagnoses.[16] Despite 3000 years of advances in medical knowledge, the earliest writings in Egypt similarly describe LBP also in 1 general diagnosis: sprain of vertebrae. Because the human back is complex, with motion and forces across tendons, muscles, bones and tissue in multiple directions, one correctly assumes that the differential diagnosis and treatment are equally as complicated. With astronomical costs to society, our treatments have not changed much over the last 3000 years.

Concerning treatment, how would you as a health care provider advise our Egyptian patient? How did the ancient healer compare with the evidence-based medicine test of today? The odds are that the ancient Egyptian physician was likely 95% accurate in his treatment. Applying today's evidence-based studies reveals that 90% to 95% of acute LBP resolves within 6 to 12 weeks regardless of our intervention.[16] It is hoped that the ancient healer did not miss any red flags (age >50 years, fever, unrelenting night pain, history of cancer, weight loss, incontinence, saddle anesthesia, progressive motor or sensory deficit, or history intravenous drug use; all of which may indicate a serious underlying condition). It seems that the ancient healer's documentation would fall short in the court of modern standards for a pertinent positive and negative history. Other observations reveal that modern medicine progressed with our recommendations for treatment regarding bed rest. We no longer recommend bed rest. Bed rest provides no benefit to patients who have acute LBP with or without sciatica. There is strong evidence that advice to stay active rather than rest in bed results in less time missed from work, less pain, and an improved functional ability.[17,18] For patients with sciatica, there is no difference in outcome between staying active versus resting in bed.[17,18] If bed rest is necessary, it should last no longer than 2 or 3 days if possible.[18]

Current treatment recommendations of LBP are covered in more detail elsewhere in this issue by Grewal and colleagues. The substantial need for care of these patients, coupled with our poor understanding of the fundamental basis of LBP in many individuals, has led to an ever-expanding array of treatment options, including medications, manual/manipulation therapy, percutaneous interventional spine procedures, and an increasing repertoire of surgical approaches.[2,19] Historically, a fair share of back pain management has been a series of expensive fads, odd contraptions, and the latest gimmicks. The high frequency of LBP mixed with the desperation of many vulnerable patients has led to easy prey for snake oil salesmen. Fertile soil for narcotic or opioid abuse has been tilled and overuse has become rampant in the past several decades, further clouding adequate treatment. Many treatments have been discredited, but not until they had been provided to scores of patients at high cost, and with occasional morbidity.[2]

Patients and health care providers are still faced with selecting from hundreds of available interventions. Although all claim to improve LBP, some often lack strong evidence to support their efficacy and safety.[16] Acute LBP with or without sciatica is usually self-limited and has no serious underlying disease.[16] For most patients, reassurance, nonnarcotic pain medications, and counseling to stay active are sufficient. Simplicity and common sense seem to guide us for much of the treatment of this disease.[16] Findings suggests an important benefit of osteopathic manipulative treatment (OMT) as a safe and cost saving treatment of LBP. Studies have demonstrated osteopathic-treatment groups verses placebo groups received less medication and less physical therapy than the "standard care" groups. Physician employing OMT demonstrated lower cost, avoided potentially serious NSAID adverse affects, and achieved equivalent outcomes in pain relief, functionality, and patient satisfaction.[20] For example, if educating and informing the patient about the natural course of the illness help, why not do it?[21] Or, in the words of the famous scientist, Albert Einstein, "Everything should be made as simple as possible, but not simpler."[22,23]

DEFINING LBP

LBP is pain localized to the lumbar area between the inferior ribcage and the waistline, although it may include sciatica, with pain radiating down the posterior-lateral thigh distal to the knee. It has commonly been divided by duration into acute (<6 weeks), subacute (6–12 weeks), and chronic (longer than 12 weeks).[16,23]

The definition of recurrent LBP is more elusive. In studies, criteria ranged from "at least 1 episode of LBP over past year" to "LBP pain twice weekly."[24,25] The variability in definitions of recurrent LBP affect the quality of research methodology and therefore the ability to translate findings into clinical practice. The cause of LBP that occurs daily for 2 weeks, daily for 2 years, or 3 times a year with or without trauma is often different. The treatment may also be different. The clinical approach to LBP is variable and if the definitions are ambiguous, multidisciplinary team communication is often adversely affected.[26]

THE PROBLEM OF LBP

LBP is common, with a peak onset at an average age of 35 years and a lifetime incidence as high as 85%.[1,16] Although 90% to 95% of cases of LBP resolve within 12 weeks, it is the most common and most expensive cause of work-related disability in the population younger than 45 years.[3] Direct medical costs because of LBP in the United States have been estimated at approximately $100 billion per year. This amount may represent only about 15% of the total cost to society, with lost productivity and disability compensation increasing the final sum.[27] Complication rates, including deaths associated with treatments for spinal pain, are also increasing, thereby increasing cost to society.[28,29]

Individuals with LBP are receiving an increasing number of interventional treatments for pain without any available evidence to support a substantial overall improvement in functional status. There is a vast and ever-expanding array of potential treatment options for LBP, many of which have some evidence of efficacy in select patients, but none of which has offered long-term benefit for most patients with LBP. There is a high patient demand for various care options for LBP, which often leaves health care professionals obligated to provide treatment recommendations based on insufficient data. The result may lead to a health care system that increasingly emphasizes the performance of narrowly focused and insufficiently studied procedures to address what are likely more complex intertwined biopsychosociospiritual-related pain problems.[30] The statistics are concerning. A lot of money is spent on more treatment options that are not effective. Evidence-based treatment protocols for the management of LBP begin to address the issue and give clinicians cost-effective quality-care guidance.[30] If we are going to identify the optimal treatment modalities for patients with LBP and show the value in our care, we must invest in high-quality outcomes research and clinical trials to determine which treatments are effective for which subsets of patients.[30]

THE SCOPE OF LBP

The epidemiology of this condition is still not well understood, and the overall prevalence of LBP in the United States remains unclear.[31] Survey data collected in 1992 and again in 2006 from a sample in North Carolina showed that the prevalence of chronic, disabling LBP rose from 3.9% of the population in 1992 to 10.2% in 2006.[32] The percentage of people who presented to physician offices for LBP based on claims-based data increased from 12% in 1998 to 15% in 2004.

Although both sets of data could suggest that the overall prevalence of LBP is increasing, it is difficult to determine to what degree these changes represent a true increase in the proportion of the population suffering from LBP or if there is an increase in diagnosis or an increase in the number of patients who report or seek medical care for LBP.[32]

THE SOCIETAL BURDEN OF LBP

Economic evaluations show that LBP remains a significant burden to the United States in terms of health care costs and employee productivity. It is estimated in the United States that the annual direct medical costs for spine problems, including LBP, doubled from $52 to $102 billion in 7 years, whereas the proportion of persons with spine problems reporting limitations in activities of daily living increased nearly 20% for the same period.[33–35]

Disability

Approximately 1% to 2% of the total US adult population are disabled because of LBP.[3,36] Self-reported health status among people with spine problems (including physical functioning, mental health, work, and social limitations) does not seem to be improving, and the overall numbers of people seeking Social Security Disability Insurance for spine-related problems and the percentage of people with disability caused by musculoskeletal pain are increasing.[33,37]

The relationship between work and LBP was recognized from the beginning of occupational medicine. In his "Treatise on the Diseases of Tradesmen," published in 1705, Ramazzini stated that servants at court who stood for long periods and weavers by the violent action of their looms were susceptible to "pains in the loyns." He noted that "the lumbago is a very common disease among laboring farmers from their frequent exposure to cold and hardships."[38] The first direct evidence of LBP disability came after the introduction of the railways. In a report "On the Influence of Railway Travel on the Public Health," the Lancet Commission gave figures showing that the amount of sickness in railway workers was greater than in mariners, miners, and laborers.[39] Railway spine became an increasing problem between 1860 and 1880.[4]

During the first 2 decades of the twentieth century, industrial back pain and low back disability became more of a widespread problem. King[40] published one of the first articles specifically about industrial back pain in 1915. Claims for LBP disability have reached epidemic numbers since 1945.

Compensation

Compensation seems to be one of the earliest social and legal characteristics of organized society. One of the earliest examples of compensation emerged in a medical negligence case. This case predates written history. The *Code of Hammurabi* (circa 1752? BC) specifically made the surgeon responsible for his action. The *Code* stated that if a slave was mortally wounded as a result of treatment, then the surgeon had to replace him. If a free man died, then the surgeon's right hand was amputated.[4]

The history of low back disability is closely linked to compensation legislation, and most modem definitions of disability imply an element of compensation. The root cause of compensation is a potential quagmire. Legislation for compensation was passed after a real need was recognized by the legal system to protect society. Compensation provides the social support that makes chronic disability possible. It is naive to deny that the prospect of receiving compensation does not attract more submission of claims. It is also cruel, unfair, and highly difficult to convict a patient of malingering within the confines of such a subjective disease. "The compensation dole has made a lazy hibernation possible."[41]

In 1861 to 1862, Henry Mayhew published *London Labor and the London Poor*. This was a 4-volume collection of oral history and reflections on interviews of some of the most destitute people. He sorted these people into 3 categories: those who can work, those who cannot work. and those who will not work. There appeared an attempt to set up a system to care for the worthy poor and mete out the unworthy poor (malingerers) through one of the first disability systems.[42]

The compensation system certainly gave us the earliest and most accurate statistics on low back disability, taking into account that noncompensated disability had not been previously recorded. There are no records of extensive low back disability claims until the 1880s and 1890s, when it was first reported in the context of compensation.[4]

Opiate Use

Several studies have discussed the growing prevalence of opioid abuse in the United States. The National Household Survey on Drug Abuse estimated that more than 6 million Americans used prescription pain relievers for nonmedical purposes in 1999. By 2001, this number had increased to 8.4 million, approximately 4% of the US population.[43]

Opioid use among persons with chronic LBP is common. The safety and efficacy of opioids for treatment of nonmalignant pain, particularly chronic LBP, is another controversial topic. Concerns regarding opioid use for chronic LBP arise from issues related to the potential for abuse, a possible lack of effectiveness, and the high rates of concurrent mental illness in those with chronic LBP. Some clinicians advocate the use of opioids in this chronic setting as a pain relief strategy, whereas others strongly oppose their use.[44] In 1 study, 12% of 20,000 individuals with back pain had received prescriptions for opioids.[45] Overall opiate use increased by 309% from 1992 to 2002 based on data from the Medicaid system in the United States.[46] A recent systematic review of opioid use for chronic pain suggested that up to 24% of patients inappropriately dose their opioid medications.[47] In addition, a meta-analysis of the available study data showed a nonsignificant difference in pain relief comparing those taking opioids and those not taking opioids.[47]

Further complicating the picture of opiate use are recent data indicating that patients taking opioids for back pain were more likely to describe underlying depression, anxiety, and other comorbid medical conditions.[48] Effective treatment of this problem often requires a multilevel approach that encompasses the full scope of comorbidities associated with chronic LBP.

SUMMARY

The diagnosis and treatment of LBP must be standardized, based on evidence and solid research. The cost to both individuals and society is great and only those diagnostic tests or treatments that can improve the quality and cost of care are advocated. The following articles review current knowledge about the neurobiology and psychology of pain perception, current pharmacology of medications used to treat pain, guidelines for the diagnosis of LBP, and various treatments used and their corresponding levels of evidence. Each article can be read alone, but in the context of the entire edition, clinicians can find current guidelines, research, and evidence-based options to manage patients with LBP.

REFERENCES

1. Bratton R. Assessment and management of acute low back pain. Am Fam Physician 1999;60:2299–308.
2. Haldeman S, Dagenais S. A supermarket approach to the evidence-informed management of chronic low back pain. Spine J 2008;8(1):1–7.
3. Deyo RA, Weinstein JN. Low back pain. N Engl J Med 2001;344(5):363–70.
4. Allen DB, Waddell G. An historical perspective on low back pain and disability. Acta Orthop Scand 1989;60(Suppl 234):1–23.
5. Knoeller SM, Seifried C. Historical perspective: history of spinal surgery. Spine 2000;25:2838–43.
6. Chedid KJ, Chedid M. The tract of history in the treatment of lumbar degenerative disc disease. Neurosurg Focus 2003;16(1):E7.
7. Keele KD. Anatomies of pain. Oxford (United Kingdom): Blackwell Scientific Publications; 1957.
8. Raether M. Psychogene Ischias. (Über psychogene. "Ischias- Rheumatismus- und Wirbelsäulenerkrankungen"). Bericht der niederrheinischen Gesellschaft für Natur– und Heilkunde in Bonn. Dtsch Med Wochenschr 1917;50:1576 [in German].
9. Mixter WJ. Rupture of the lumbar intervertebral disk. Ann Surg 1937;106:777–87.
10. Barr JS. Lumbar disk in retrospect and prospect. Clin Orthop 1977;129:4–8.
11. Boden SD, Davis OD, Dina TS. Abnormal magnetic resonance scans of the lumbar spine in asymptomatic subjects. J Bone Joint Surg 1990;3:403–8.
12. Enzmann DR. On low back pain. AJNR Am J Neuroradiol 1994;15:109–13.
13. Lutz G, Butzlaff M, Schultz-Venrath U, et al. Looking back on back pain: trial and error of the diagnosis in the 20th century. Spine (Phila Pa 1976) 2003;28(16):1899–905.
14. Deyo RA. Rethinking strategies for acute low back pain. Acad Emerg Med 1994; 11:38–56.
15. Raspe H. A database for back (axial skeletal) pain. Rheum Dis Clin North Am 1995;21:559–79.
16. Kincade S. Evaluation and treatment of acute low back pain. Am Fam Physician 2007;75(8):1181–8.
17. Hagen KB, Hilde G, Jamtvedt G, et al. Bed rest for acute low-back pain and sciatica. Cochrane Database Syst Rev 2004;(4):CD001254.
18. Hilde G, Hagen KB, Jamtvedt G, et al. Advice to stay active as a single treatment for low back pain and sciatica. Cochrane Database Syst Rev 2006;(2):CD003632.
19. Deyo RA, Mirza SK, Turner JA, et al. Overtreating chronic back pain: time to back off? J Am Board Fam Med 2009;22(1):62–8.
20. Andersson GBJ, Lucente T, Davis AM, et al. A Comparison of Osteopathic spinal manipulation with standard care for patients with low back pain. The New England Journal of Medicine 1999;341(19).
21. Boden SD, Dreyer SJ, Levy HI. Management of low back pain. Current assessment and the formulation of a blueprint for the health care delivery. Phys Med Rehabil Clin North Am 1998;9(2):419–33.
22. Einstein A. Readers Digest 1977.
23. Duffy L. Low back pain: an approach to diagnosis and management. Prim Care 2010;37:729–41.
24. Bruce B, Lorig K, Laurent D, et al. The impact of a moderated e-mail discussion group on use of complementary and alternative therapies in subjects with recurrent back pain. Patient Educ Couns 2005;58:305–11.
25. Feuerstein M, Carter RL, Papciak AS, et al. A prospective analysis of stress and fatigue in recurrent low back pain. Pain 1987;31:333–44.

26. Stanton T. How do we define the condition 'recurrent low back pain'? A systematic review. Eur Spine J 2010;19:533–9.

27. Dagenais S, Caro J, Haldeman S. A systematic review of low back pain cost of illness studies in the United States and internationally. Spine J 2008;8(1):8–20.

28. Bigos SJ, Bowyer OR, Braen GR, et al. Acute low back problems in adults. Clinical practice guideline no. 14 (AHCPR publication no. 95–0642). Rockville (MD): Department of Health and Human Services, Public Health Service, Agency for Health Care Policy and Research; 1994.

29. Last A, Hulbert K. Chronic low back pain: evaluation and management. Am Fam Physician 2009;79(12):1067–74.

30. Friedly J, Standaert C, Chan L. Epidemiology of spine care: the back pain dilemma. Phys Med Rehabil Clin North Am 2010;21(4):659–77.

31. Bone and Joint Decade. In: Katz S, editor. The burden of musculoskeletal diseases in the United States. Rosemont (IL): American Academy of Orthopaedic Surgeons; 2008.

32. Freburger JK, Holmes GM, Agans RP, et al. The rising prevalence of chronic low back pain. Arch Intern Med 2009;169(3):251–8.

33. Martin BI, Deyo RA, Mirza SK, et al. Expenditures and health status among adults with back and neck problems. JAMA 2008;299:656–64.

34. Dagenais S, Caro J, Haldeman S. Escalation of cost. Spine J 2009;9:944–57.

35. Asche CV. The societal costs of low back pain. J Pain Palliat Care Pharmacother 2007;21(4):25–43.

36. Anderson G. The epidemiology of spinal disorders. In: Frymoyer JW, editor. The adult spine: principles and practice. 2nd edition. Philadelphia: Lippincott-Raven; 1997.

37. Weiner DK, Kim YS, Bonino P, et al. Low back pain in older adults: are we utilizing healthcare resources wisely? Pain Med 2006;7(2):143–50.

38. Fowler T. Medical reports of the effects of blood letting, sudorifics and blistering in the cure of acute and chronic rheumatism. London: Johnstone; 1795.

39. Lancet Commission. The influence of railway travelling on public health. Hardwicke; 1862. p. 15–9, 48–53, 79–84.

40. Waddell G. A new clinical model for the treatment of low back pain. Spine 1987; 12:632–44.

41. Osgood RB, Momson LB. The problem of the industrial lame back. Boston Med Surg J 1924;191:381–91.

42. Hadler N. The disabling back. Spine 1995;20(6):640–9.

43. Sikka R, Xia F, Aubert RE. Estimating medication persistency using administrative claims data. J Manag Care Pharm 2005;11(7):449–57.

44. Mahowald ML, Singh JA, Majeski P. Opioid use by patients in an orthopedics spine clinic. Arthritis Rheum 2005;52(1):312–21.

45. Luo X, Pietrobon R, Sun SX, et al. Estimates and patterns of direct health care expenditures among individuals with low back pain in the United States. Spine 2004;29:79–86.

46. Zerzan JT, Morden NE, Soumerai S, et al. Trends and geographic variation of opiate medication use in state Medicaid fee-for-service programs, 1996 to 2002. Med Care 2006;44(11):1005–10.

47. Martell BA, O'Connor PG, Kerns RD, et al. Systematic review: opioid treatment for chronic back pain: prevalence, efficacy, and association with addiction. Ann Intern Med 2007;146(2):116–27.

48. Rhee Y, Taitel MS, Walker DR, et al. Narcotic drug use among patients with lower back pain in employer health plans: a retrospective analysis of risk factors and health care services. Clin Ther 2007;29(Suppl):2603–12.

Evaluation and Diagnosis of Low Back Pain

Eron G. Manusov, MD

KEYWORDS

- Low back pain • Evaluation • Diagnosis • Clinical decision making

KEY POINTS

- The diagnosis of low back pain is complicated by the varying presentations and complex nature of pain and the nonstandardized approach by physicians to clinical decision making.
- Despite the existence of at least 10 national or international guidelines available to assist with clinical decision making, only 29% of physicians use any guideline to diagnose low back pain.[1–3]
- Although there is controversy about which diagnostic algorithm primary care physicians should use, it is clear that most causes of low back pain are a result of mechanical forces and quickly resolve without costly imaging. Physicians should rely on the history and physical examination and look for medical red flags that point to serious or life-threatening causes of low back pain.

The diagnosis of low back pain is complicated by the varying presentations and complex nature of pain and the nonstandardized approach by physicians to clinical decision making. Despite the existence of at least 10 national or international guidelines available to assist with clinical decision making, only 29% of physicians use any guideline to make the diagnosis of low back pain.[1–3] It is unclear why physicians do not use guidelines to establish the diagnosis of low back pain. Possible reasons may include: low back pain is complicated by diverse multifactorial cause and presentation scenarios, there is a complex psychosocial overlay in low back pain, and there is a diversity of outcomes. More importantly, there is a paucity of evidence-based scientific information to support any 1 clinical decision-making tool.

The purpose of this article is to review the evidence available for the diagnosis of low back pain and present a cost-effective and reasonable evidence-based approach to the diagnosis of low back pain. Other articles elsewhere in this issue review evidence for various treatment options, including both neurologic and cognitive control modalities. A correct diagnosis that is broad enough to consider a differential diagnosis but focused enough to contain unnecessary costs greatly simplifies treatment and management of low back pain.

Southern Regional Area Health Education Center (SR-AHEC), 1601 Owens Drive, Fayetteville, NC 28304, USA
E-mail address: Eron.manusov@sr-ahec.org

Prim Care Clin Office Pract 39 (2012) 471–479
http://dx.doi.org/10.1016/j.pop.2012.06.003
0095-4543/12/$ – see front matter © 2012 Elsevier Inc. All rights reserved.

BACKGROUND

Low back pain is a common musculoskeletal condition, with considerable associated disability, work absenteeism, health care costs, and burden to US society. It has been estimated that 85% of adults suffer from low back pain at some time during their lives.[1–3] The usual age of onset is between 30 and 50 years and is the most common cause of work-related disability among Americans younger than 45 years.[4] Women are slightly more likely to report back pain (28% vs 24.3% level of evidence [LOE] B, low-quality randomized controlled trial [RCT]) than men.[4] Most (30%–60%) patients recover within 1 week of onset of pain. Up to 90% recover within 6 weeks. Most individuals do not seek medical care to treat their pain. As many as 50% of patients with back pain report recurrence of pain within 6 months, and up to 33% of patients report at least a moderate level of intensity of pain up to 1 year after an acute episode of low back pain.[3,5] With only 25% to 30% of patients not seeking medical care, and most improving within 6 weeks, it is surprising that low back pain accounts for 2% of all physician office visits. Low back pain is the fifth most common reason cited for visiting a health care provider.[5] The inflation-adjusted medical cost for treating low back pain increased from 1997 to 2005 by 60%.[6] It has been estimated that in 2005 the treatment of low back pain added a cost of 85.9 billion dollars to the US health care system.

MULTIFACTORIAL CAUSE OF LOW BACK PAIN

The low back is defined as the lumbar region from the inferior border of the thoracic rib cage to the sacrum. There are 5 lumbar vertebrae, each with a load-bearing central body. The pedicles and lamina extend from the body and support 2 transverse processes and a single spinous process. The intervertebral disk separates the vertebral bodies and acts as a shock absorber. The nucleus pulposus, a remnant of the embryonic notochord, is more viscoelastic, centrally positioned, and is not innervated. The surrounding outer ring of innervated, elastic collagen provides for more structured support. Pressure and wear and tear result in less elastic fibrous tissue, which replaces the elastic collagen. This situation leads to signs and symptoms of disk degeneration. If the pressure is great enough, the central nucleus pulposus may extrude and irritate the exiting nerve root. Pain can arise from the innervated intervertebral disk, the facet joint, paravertebral muscles, ligaments, and fascia (**Fig. 1**).

As shown in **Fig. 2** the vertebra can be pictured as 2 cans separated by a donut, with the complex itself surrounded by duct tape. When the donut is fresh, there is little motion of the 2 cans. As the donut hardens there is decreased support and decreased absorptive capacity. Should the jelly squish out of the donut there is increased multidirectional motion of the cans (**Fig. 2**B). Using this analogy it is easy to see why only 15% of patients with low back pain have a specific identifiable cause of pain.[7] Increased motion, decreased cushioning, degeneration and abnormal bone formation, and degeneration and weakening of muscles and ligaments can cause pain at any of the multiple articulations and innervated structures.

CLASSIFICATION STRATEGIES

Low back pain can be classified by several categories. There is no one classification system that is better for the categorization of low back pain. In a meta-analysis that reviewed 60 articles on chronic low back pain, 28 articles met inclusion criteria and were critically evaluated. In addition to flaws in methodology and statistics, some were descriptive, some prognostic, and some attempted to direct treatment. The

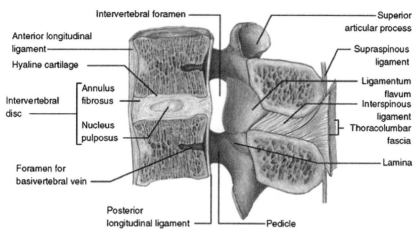

Fig. 1. The anatomy of the lumbar vertebra. (*From* Putz R, Pabst R. Sobotta atlas of human anatomy: thorax, abdomen, pelvis, lower limb. 14th edition. Vol. 2. London: Churchill Livingstone; 2006; with permission.)

recommendation of the investigators was that no one classification system be adopted for all approaches (LOE B low-quality RCT).[8]

However, a classification should assist with the formation of a differential diagnosis. **Table 1** divides the causes of low back pain into 3 categories: mechanical, nonmechanical, and visceral causes for low back pain. Ninety-seven percent of cases of low back pain fall into the musculoskeletal or mechanical causes of pain. Only 1% of patients have a nonmusculoskeletal or nonmechanical cause of low back pain and 2% have a visceral cause of low back pain. The benefit of using the differential diagnosis to evaluate low back pain is that 97% of low back pain falls in the category of mechanical and therefore the evaluation can focus on the major causes of pain.

Another classification listed in **Tables 2** and **3** is based on signs and symptoms. The 3 categories are nonspecific low back pain, radicular back pain, and worrisome or medical red flags. Nonspecific low back pain is the most common (85%). The pain emanates from ligaments, tendons, muscles, and nerve fibers around the vertebra and its articulations. The pain may radiate to the buttocks, but not below the knee.

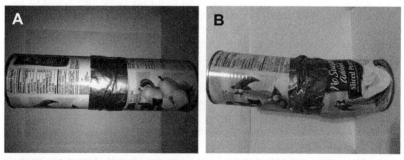

Fig. 2. The 2 cans, 1 jelly donut, and duct tape model of lumbar vertebra. (*A*) If the jelly donut is full, the 2 cans are held together with tight duct tape and there is little motion. (*B*) If the jelly donut is depleted, the 2 cans are held together with loose duct tape and there is a lot of motion.

Table 1
Classification of low back pain by categories and differential diagnosis

Mechanical Low Back Pain (90%)	Nonmechanical Low Back Pain	Visceral Disease
Musculoskeletal strain 1. Ligament 2. Muscle 3. Fascia 4. Pregnancy and posterior pelvic ring pain	Neoplasm 1. Multiple myeloma 2. Lymphoma and leukemia 3. Spinal cord tumors 4. Retroperitoneal tumors 5. Osteoma	Diseases of pelvic organs 1. Prostatis 2. Endometriosis 3. Chronic pelvic Inflammatory disease
Herniated disk 1. Herniated nucleus pulposus 2. Impingement of exiting nerves	Infection 1. Osteomyelitis 2. Diskitis 3. Epidural or paraspinous abscess 4. Tuberculosis 5. Shingles	Renal disease 1. Nephrolithiasis 2. Pyelonephritis 3. Perinephric abscess
Diskogenic causes of pain 1. Replacement of elastic tissue with fibrous tissue 2. Tears and degeneration of disk	Inflammatory arthritis (HLAB27) 1. Ankylosing spondylitis 2. Psoriatic spondylitis 3. Reiter syndrome 4. Inflammatory bowel disease	Vascular 1. Aortic aneurysm
Facet degeneration 1. Degeneration and calcification of facet joint 2. Decreased motion of facet joint	Scheuermann disease (osteochondrosis)	Gastrointestinal disease 1. Pancreatitis 2. Cholecystitis 3. Penetrating ulcer
Spinal stenosis	Paget disease	
Spondylolisthesis/ spondylolitholysis	Sickle cell anemia	
Scoliosis >25°		
Osteoporotic fracture		

Radicular or sciatic pain occurs in 7% of patients with low back pain. Pain radiates below the knee and if bilateral, usually indicates spinal stenosis. Unilateral pain is associated with the L5 and S1 nerve roots in 95% of cases. The third category includes medical red flags, or those diagnoses that may need immediate or specific treatment such as tumor, infection, visceral causes, cauda equina syndrome, ankylosing spondylitis or spondylolisthesis, and compression fracture. The benefit to the classification listed in **Table 2** is that evaluation and treatment can be focused on the dangerous or immediate diagnoses that need to be approached immediately. Pressure on an exiting nerve root by a herniated disk can result in atrophy of the innervated muscle and therefore permanent neurologic deficit. Treatment results in variable success. Because the diagnosis is most times multifactorial in cause, specific focused treatment is variable in success. Once the medical red flags are ruled out, the most effective treatment can be multimodal and directed at a presumed radicular or nonradicular cause.

It is helpful to distinguish between acute and chronic causes of low back pain. Acute pain is defined as immediate and lasting less than 6 weeks. Chronic pain is pain that lasts longer than 3 months.[9] The period between 6 weeks and 3 months is referred to subacute pain. In the subacute period, acute pain has the potential to become chronic

Table 2
Classification of low back pain by signs and symptoms

Nonspecific Low Back Pain (85%)	Radicular (7%)	Worrisome Red Flags
Radiates to buttocks	Pain radiates below the knee	Major trauma
Diffuse pain	Unilateral (disk herniation)	Age >50 y
No specific maneuver to increase or reduce pain	Bilateral (spinal stenosis)	Persistent fever
	Worse with sitting	History of cancer
	Improves with lying and knees bent to reduce tension on sciatic nerve	Metabolic disorder
		Major muscle weakness
		Saddle anesthesia
		Decreased sphincter tone
		Unrelenting night pain

pain. Acute pain is based on nocioceptive receptors or neuropathic receptors. As pain becomes more chronic, the pain patterns become more complex, with various bio-psychosocial components. Pain reception and perception are discussed in 2 articles elsewhere in this issue because of the complexity of central nervous system biologic changes such as neuronal hyperexcitability, membrane changes, gene expression, and pathway formation. Cognitive, social, emotional, and psychological changes further complicate diagnosis and management.

DIAGNOSTIC APPROACH TO LOW BACK PAIN
History

A thorough patient history is important in the evaluation of low back pain. Clinicians can approach the differential diagnosis of low back pain and determine if there are any medical red flags or cause that needs immediate or specific intervention.[10] **Box 1** lists historical red flags. The clinician tries to answer the following 3 questions:

1. Is there a neurologic deficit that may require surgical intervention?
2. Is there a systemic disease or cancer that can be causing the pain?
3. Are there other factors that may complicate the diagnosis or treatment?

The first 2 questions do not help to differentiate between mechanical or musculo-skeletal causes of back pain. The answers help determine if further consultation, such as with a surgeon or oncologist, is necessary. The third question helps determine if there are complicating situations that may affect eventual outcome. For example, a patient may be depressed, be in litigation, desire disability insurance, be involved in opioid diversion, or suffer from mental illness.

Initial Assessment of Acute Low Back Pain

In the absence of red flags, diagnostic testing is not clinically helpful in the first 4 weeks of symptoms.[5] If medical red flags are present, further investigation for spinal fracture, cancer or infection, cauda equina syndrome, or rapidly progressing neurologic deficit must occur. Older patients with signs of osteoporosis are susceptible to compression fractures; younger patients may describe pain on lateral back bend with a pars

Table 3
Risk factors or red flags identified on history or physical examination can direct imaging

Mechanical Low Back Pain (90%)	Imaging	Nonmechanical Low Back Pain (1%)	Imaging	Visceral Disease (2%)	Imaging
Musculoskeletal strain 1. Ligament 2. Muscle 3. Fascia 4. Pregnancy and posterior pelvic ring pain	N/A	Neoplasm 1. Multiple myeloma 2. Lymphoma and leukemia 3. Spinal cord tumors 4. Retroperitoneal tumors 5. Retroperitoneal tumors 6. Osteoma	Plain films MRI Radionuclide	Diseases of pelvic organs 1. Prostatis 2. Endometriosis 3. Chronic pelvic inflammatory disease	N/A
Herniated disk 1. Herniated nucleus pulposus 2. Impingement of exiting nerves	MRI	Infection 1. Osteomyelitis 2. Diskitis 3. Epidural or paraspinous abscess 4. Shingles	Plain films MRI	Renal disease 1. Nephrolithiasis 2. Pyelonephritis 3. Perinephric abscess	Intravenous pyelography Ultrasonography
Diskogenic causes of pain 1. Replacement of elastic tissue with fibrous tissue 2. Tears and degeneration of disk	MRI	Inflammatory arthritis (HLAB27) 1. Ankylosing spondylitis 2. Psoriatic spondylitis 3. Reiter syndrome 4. Inflammatory bowel disease	Plain films CT scan	Vascular 1. Aortic aneurysm	Ultrasonography MRI with contrast
Facet degeneration 1. Degeneration and calcification of facet joint 2. Decreased motion of facet joint	Plain films MRI CT scan	Scheuermann disease (osteochondrosis)	Plain films	Gastrointestinal disease 1. Pancreatitis 2. Cholecystitis 3. Penetrating ulcer	Plain films
Spinal stenosis	CT and MRI equal	Paget disease			
Spondylolisthesis/spondylolitholysis	Plain films				
Scoliosis >25°	Plain films				
Osteoporotic fracture	Plain films				

Adapted from Jarvik JG, Deyo RA. Diagnostic evaluation of low back pain with emphasis on imaging. Ann Intern Med 2002;137:556.

Box 1
Historical medical red flags in the diagnosis of low back pain

1. Age less than 20 years or greater than 50 years

2. History of intravenous drug use

3. History of cancer

4. Constitutional signs such as fever, chills, nausea, or weight loss

5. Saddle anesthesia/bowel or bladder incontinence/retention

6. Recent bacterial infection

7. Unrelenting nocturnal pain/pain increased in the supine position

8. History of immune suppression

9. History of chronic steroid use

10. History of recent trauma

11. History of tuberculosis

---

interarticularis fracture; a patient with history of prostate symptoms may describe pain caused by metastatic prostate cancer. A patient with ankylosing spondylitis may describe early morning stiffness, early morning waking because of pain, and pain that improves with exercise. There is usually a family history of ankylosing spondylitis.

The clinician should then further define the nature of the pain. The history should include onset of pain, duration of pain, location of pain, severity of pain, triggers of pain, and associated signs and symptoms of pain. Other questions include those directed at motor loss, sensory loss, bladder or bowel incontinence/retention, and past treatment. More specific to children are leukemia and sickle cell disease presenting as back pain.[10]

A focused physical examination should concentrate on the differential diagnosis to include nonback or visceral causes of back pain such as pancreatitis, nephrolithiasis, and aortic aneurysm. Systemic illness including endocarditis, viral syndromes, Pott disease (tuberculosis), sickle cell anemia, and cancer all have characteristic physical findings. Localized infection such as epidural abscess, transverse myelitis, osteomyelitis, diskitis, and syphilis can also present as back pain. The neurologic examination can define a level of deficit by sensory or motor findings. Sitting and lying straight leg lifts can stretch an irritated sciatic nerve. Examinations can focus on the iliopsoas muscle or tendon, the sacroiliac joint, and the pyriformis muscle. Urinary retention has a 90% sensitivity to diagnose cauda equina syndrome.[11,12]

In a Cochrane review of 16 cohort studies (median N = 126; range 71–2504) and 3 case control students (38–100 cases), most physical tests show low sensitivity and specificity. In a surgical population characterized by high prevalence of disk herniation (58%–98%), the straight leg raise showed a high sensitivity (pooled estimate 0.92; 95% confidence interval, 0.87–0.95). Otherwise, when used in isolation, diagnostic performance on most physical tests (scoliosis, paresis, muscle weakness, muscle wasting, impaired reflexes, and sensory deficits) was poor.[13]

Radiographs and Low Back Pain

Routine roentgenographs for low back pain without red flags are not indicated. Low back pain is often multifactorial and related to mechanical or nonspecific causes. Plain roentgenographs or advanced imaging such as magnetic resonance imaging (MRI) and computed tomography (CT) are not value added to the early management of patients.[11] Because many patients with or without low back pain have abnormalities on imaging tests, false-positive results can cause increased anxiety, increased spending, and increased procedures. Physicians often quote fear of lawsuits or missed diagnosis as reasons to order early roentgenographs. The American College of Physicians recommendations help to standardize care and therefore support careful waiting and conservative care.

For low back pain with red flags, imaging is indicated. In addition, failure to improve, deterioration of symptoms, persistent neurologic deficit, or change of nature of the pain can signify a cause worse than musculoskeletal pain. Radiography with a posterior anterior (PA), lateral, and oblique radiograph are sufficient to see most mechanical causes of low back pain (**Fig. 3**A, B). Risk factors or red flags identified on history or physical examination can direct imaging.[10]

In a meta-analysis published in 2002, the investigators determined that MRI had the highest sensitivity for the detection of cancer at 0.83 to 0.93, with specificity of 0.9 to 0.97. Bone scan sensitivity for the detection of cancer was 0.74 to 0.98 and the highest specificity for cancer detection was plain radiography (0.95 to 0.99). For infection, MRI was most sensitive (0.96) and specific for infection (0.92).[11] For herniated disks, MRI had a slightly higher sensitivity than CT but both techniques were similar for the diagnosis of spinal stenosis.[14]

More advanced imaging is required for severe or persistent neurologic deficit or for red flags characteristic of poor prognosis without intervention.[14,15] Infections, cancers, and cauda equina syndrome require earlier imagining techniques. Otherwise, watchful waiting and alternative treatment regimens decrease unnecessary interventions and decrease health care dollars spent on a common problem.

There is evidence for diagnostic procedures such as facet joint blocks and transforaminal epidural injections. There is strong evidence for the diagnostic accuracy of

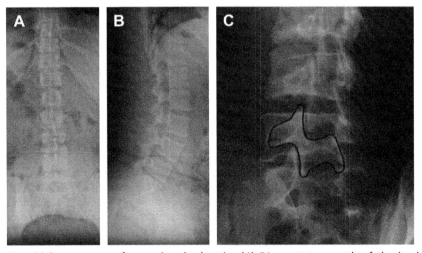

Fig. 3. Initial assessment of acute low back pain. (*A*) PA roentgenograph of the lumbar sacral spine series. (*B*) Lateral roentgenograph of the lumbar sacral spine series. (*C*) Oblique roentgenograph of the lumbar sacral spine series with Scotty dog sign. (*From* Glassman SD, Carreon LY, Anderson PA, et al. A diagnostic classification for lumbar spine registry development. Spine J. 2011 Dec;11(12):1114 [*A,B*]; and Maxfield BA. Sports-related injury of the pediatric spine. Radiol Clin North Am 48(6):1244 [*C*]; with permission.)

facet joint blocks in evaluating spinal pain, and moderate evidence for transforaminal epidural injections. Sacroiliac injections can also be helpful for diagnosis. Pain reduction with anesthetic injection can support a specific anatomic source.

Although there is controversy about which diagnostic algorithm primary care physicians should use, it is clear that most low back pain is caused by mechanical forces and quickly resolves without costly imaging. Physicians should rely on the history and physical examination and look for medical red flags that point to serious or life-threatening causes of low back pain.

REFERENCES

1. Dagenais S, Tricco AC, Haldemann S. Synthesis of recommendations for the assessment and management of low back pain from recent clinical practice guidelines. Spine J 2010;10(6):514–29.
2. Chou R, Quaseem A, Snow V. Diagnosis and treatment of low back pain: a joint clinical practice guideline for the American College of Physicians and the American Pain Society. Ann Intern Med 2007;1447:478–91.
3. Chou R, Loeser JD, Owens DK, American Pain Society Low Back Pain Guideline Panel. Interventional therapies, surgery, and interdisciplinary rehabilitation for low back pain: an evidence based clinical practice guideline from the American Pain Society. Spine 2009;34(10):1066–77.
4. Deyo RA, Mirza SK, Martin BL. Back pain prevalence and visit rates: estimates from U.S. national surveys. Spine 2001;2006(31):2724–7.
5. Kinkade S. Evaluation and treatment of acute low back pain. Am Fam Physician 2007;75:1181–8.
6. Martin BI, Deyo RA, Mirza SK. Expenditures and health status among adults with back and neck problems. JAMA 2008;299(6):656–64.
7. Available at: http://wwwmed-iq/a587. Accessed February 9, 2012.
8. Frymoyer JW. Back pain and sciatica. N Engl J Med 1988;318:291–300.
9. Fairbank J, Qwilym SE, France JC, et al. The role of classification of chronic low back pain. Spine (Phila Pa 1976) 2011;36(Suppl 21):S19–42.
10. Focused History Tool. 10 Available at: http://med-iq.com/s36. Accessed February 9, 2012.
11. Available at: http://www.icsi.org/low_back_pain/adult_low_back_pain__8.html. Accessed February 9, 2012.
12. Jarvic JG, Deyo RA. Diagnostic evaluation of low back pain with emphasis on imaging. Ann Intern Med 2002;137:556.
13. van der Windt DA, Simons E, Riphagen II, et al. Physical examination for lumbar radiculopathy due to disc herniation in patients with low-back pain. Cochrane Database Syst Rev 2010;(2):CD007431.
14. Chaou R, Qaseem A, Owens DK, et al, Clinical Guidelines Committee of the American College of Physicians. Diagnostic imaging for low back pain: advice for high-value health care from the American College of Physicians. Ann Intern Med 2011;154(3):181–9.
15. Rubinstein SM, van Tulder M. A best-evidence review of diagnostic procedures for neck and low-back pain. Best Pract Res Clin Rheumatol 2008;22(3):471–82.

Treatment: Current Treatment Recommendations for Acute and Chronic Undifferentiated Low Back Pain

Rebekah Sprouse, MD

KEYWORDS

- Low back pain • Recommendations • Joint clinical practice guideline

KEY POINTS

- In 2007, the American College of Physicians and the American Pain Society formed the Clinical Efficacy Assessment Subcommittee to reassess the recommendations for the diagnosis and treatment of low back pain. The recommendations were published in the Annals of Internal Medicine. These guidelines were based on 2 main foundations: (1) most low back pain improves without intervention, and (2) although the history and physical are the cornerstones of management, costly radiologic evaluation of patients with low back pain was still popular in 2007.
- The differential for low back pain can be divided into 3 major subsets: (1) back pain that is not related to a neurologic problem, (2) back pain related to a problem with the spinal column, or (3) back pain related to another neurologic issue. In addition to separating back pain into 1 of these 3 categories, pain can also be classified as acute versus chronic.
- For patients with low back pain who are not currently on any type of therapy, the first-line treatment is self-care and continued activity, because bed rest can worsen the prognosis for acute low back pain.

This article is an overview of current treatment recommendations for low back pain, and includes recommendations from the Joint Clinical Practice Guideline from the American College of Physicians and the American Pain Society. As discussed elsewhere in this issue by Maharty and colleagues, back pain is common and costly. Often, it does not require medical treatment because it resolves on its own, but, for patients who do require treatment, the effective management of the pain, disability, and psychosocial aspects of the condition can mean the difference between a quick return to function and lifelong disability.

Southern Regional Area Health Education Center, 1601 Owen Drive, Fayetteville, NC 28304, USA
E-mail address: rebekah.Sprouse@sr-ahec.org

Prim Care Clin Office Pract 39 (2012) 481–486
http://dx.doi.org/10.1016/j.pop.2012.06.004   **primarycare.theclinics.com**
0095-4543/12/$ – see front matter © 2012 Elsevier Inc. All rights reserved.

In 1994, the US Agency for Health Care Policy and Research released practice guidelines regarding treatment of low back pain.[1] The recommendations published were controversial because the standard of care was primarily surgical. However, the recommendations were based on research that supported the concept of recovery without surgical intervention. Patient education and modalities designed to improve comfort were emphasized in the 1994 practice guidelines. These recommendations included the use of over-the-counter medications such as acetaminophen or nonsteroidal antiinflammatory drugs (NSAIDs) with progression to short-term opioid use only if necessary. Muscle relaxants had no greater benefit than NSAIDs and were therefore not recommended. If simple medical therapies were determined to be inadequate, physical modalities such as basic physical therapy with heat or cold, and noninvasive methods such as traction, massage, shoe lifts, biofeedback, cutaneous laser treatment, and transcutaneous electrical nerve stimulators were recommended. Invasive treatments, including acupuncture and steroid injections, were recommended despite the lack of research documenting any substantial benefit for either intervention.[1]

In 2007, the American College of Physicians and the American Pain Society formed the Clinical Efficacy Assessment Subcommittee to reassess the recommendations for the diagnosis and treatment of low back pain. The recommendations were published in the *Annals of Internal Medicine*.[2] These guidelines were based on 2 main foundations: (1) most low back pain improves without intervention, and (2) although the history and physical is the cornerstone of management, costly radiologic evaluation of patients with low back pain was still popular in 2007. The 2007 recommendations de-emphasized radiologic evaluations, a holdover from the 1990s, and stressed the importance of a careful comprehensive history and physical examination, recognition of red flags or warning signs, and a progressive approach to diagnostic imaging and treatment.[2]

Despite advances in research and evidence-based guidelines, the diagnosis and management of low back pain remains controversial. From anatomic and neurologic standpoints, the low back is complicated, which makes diagnosis difficult. From a biologic perspective, pain is a subjective experience that is multifactorial in cause and is exacerbated by the interrelated psychosocial correlates that affect a patient's experience (eg, culture, finances, perception, emotional distress). In addition, systemic and societal issues such as law suits, disability compensation, and a health care system that offers rewards for more procedures and expensive diagnostic techniques further complicate and influence the diagnosis and management of low back pain.

A MODEL FOR TREATMENT AND DIAGNOSIS

To better understand the 7 recommendations from 2007 it is necessary to review a differential diagnosis of low back pain that is divided into categories (**Fig. 1**). As reviewed elsewhere in this issue, the differential for low back pain can be divided into 3 major subsets: (1) back pain that is not related to a neurologic problem, (2) back pain related to a problem with the spinal column, or (3) back pain related to another neurologic issue.[1] These categories can help predict, by generalizing the source or cause of the pain with stratification into likelihood of resolution, the likelihood of the patient's back pain progressing to a chronic or debilitating condition. Information regarding categorization should come from a history and physical that is detailed specifically for back pain, but still broad enough to include possible reasons for back pain, such as malignancy or infection. The categories allow subsequent tests and to be guided and imaging to be as efficient as possible, and also limit the risk of misdiagnosis that could lead to lifelong disability or, in some cases, death (aortic aneurysm rupture). In addition to separating back pain into 1 of these 3 categories, pain can also

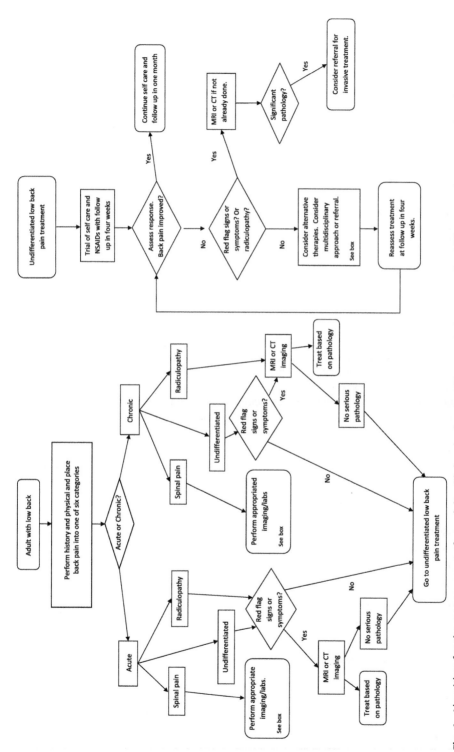

Fig. 1. Algorithm for the management of an adult with low back pain. CT, computed tomography; MRI, magnetic resonance imaging.

be classified as acute versus chronic. Although useful to help guide treatment options, the classification of acute versus chronic pain can also help with developing a more accurate differential diagnosis, and gives a more accurate prognosis for the patient regarding recovery.

Acute versus Chronic

Acute back pain lasts from a few days to a few weeks, however, in most cases, it resolves with or without treatment in 4 weeks. Those who do not recover in the first 4 weeks generally see marked improvement in the first 3 months. The differential diagnosis for acute or sudden low back pain can include, but is not limited to, muscle spasm, fracture, sciatica, or stenosis.[2] It is also important to evaluate the patient immediately for signs considered to be red flags that make back pain an emergency, such as incontinence of stool or urine, signs of vertebral infection, or sudden weakness in an extremity listed in **Box 1**. If any of these signs are present, further evaluation is indicated. It is also important to evaluate for psychosocial risk factors, such as coping behaviors, overall functional status, general health, as well as psychosocial comorbidities and mental health. The more psychosocial risk factors involved, the more likely the patient will develop chronic back pain and progress to long-term disability. In contrast, early intervention that addresses these psychosocial issues may improve the likelihood of complete and early recovery.

Chronic back pain is defined as pain that has lasted more than 3 months, and can include the patient with untreated back pain and the patient with failed acute back pain treatment. The patient with chronic back pain must also be evaluated for red flag signs because these signs and symptoms can develop over long periods of time, or can be seen with acute exacerbations of chronic back pain. The development of chronic back pain can be more insidious in that it can begin by being manageable, but have a slowly progressive increase in the level of pain. Possible diagnoses for chronic pain are similar to those for acute back pain, although the pain is less likely to be caused by trauma and more to have a diagnosis such as cancer, with the pain stemming from fracture secondary to tumor growth.[2]

Box 1
Red flags, or signs and symptoms that may indicate a serious cause of low back pain

Red flags for back pain

Age more than 50 years

History of cancer

Unexplained weight loss

Persistent fever

History of intravenous drug use

Immunocompromised state

Recent bacterial infection

Urinary or stool incontinence

Urinary retention

Extremity weakness

Neurologic deficit

Trauma

Approximately 85% of patients who present to a primary care physician have back pain that cannot be attributed to a specific diagnosis.[1] If no neurologic source of back pain is diagnosed and there are no red flag symptoms, the patient is diagnosed with nonspecific low back pain. This type of back pain does not require any type of special imaging. At this point, treatment options should be discussed with the patient along with the goal of each option.

If a consensus is not achieved between the physician and the patient, it will be difficult to achieve a successful result.

Treatment

For patients with low back pain who are not currently on any type of therapy, the first-line treatment is self-care and continued activity, because bed rest can worsen the prognosis for acute low back pain (**Box 2**). Short periods of rest may be necessary for patients with severe pain, but these should be kept to a minimum; patients should be encouraged to continue with daily activities.[1] In addition, stretching exercises, as recommended in a book or simple printed handouts provided by the clinic, added to management will improve the course of recovery. If the back pain is acute, application of heat can also be helpful for temporary relief of pain.[1]

Box 2
Initial treatment of low back pain

Low back pain therapy[a]

Self-care

    Remain active

    Stretching exercises

    Superficial heat

Pharmacologic therapy

    Acetaminophen

    NSAIDs

    Skeletal muscle relaxants

    Tricyclic antidepressants

    Benzodiazepines

    Tramadol, opioids

Alternative therapies

    Spinal manipulation

    Exercise therapy

    Massage

    Acupuncture

    Yoga

    Cognitive behavior therapy

    Progressive relaxation

Multidisciplinary rehabilitation

[a] Level of evidence is variable.

An appointment for reevaluation should be scheduled with the patient in 4 weeks to assess improvement. Patients who experience improvement should be followed for 1 additional month. If the patient does not improve on the self-care therapy, the diagnosis should be reconsidered, and the patient should be thoroughly examined once again and questioned for red flag symptoms. At this point, the need for imaging should be readdressed as well.[2]

Patients not meeting criteria for a diagnosis other than nonspecific low back pain should be considered for pharmacologic and additional nonpharmocologic therapy in addition to continuing self-care. For acute back pain, management includes acetaminophen, NSAIDs, skeletal muscle relaxants, benzodiazepines, tramadol, opioids, and spinal manipulation. Patients with chronic low back pain should be considered for acetaminophen, NSAIDs, benzodiazepines, tramadol, opioids, and spinal manipulation, as well as additional nonpharmacologic treatments such as acupuncture, massage therapy, yoga, exercise therapy, cognitive behavior therapy, and progressive relaxation (see **Box 2**). After initiation of 1 or more of these therapies, follow-up should again be in 4 weeks (strong recommendation, moderate-quality evidence).[3,4] If there is improvement or resolution of symptoms, treatment should be continued and an additional 1 month reevaluation appointment should be scheduled. However, if no benefit has been reported with these therapies, referral to an intensive interdisciplinary rehabilitation center may be needed.

Although treating back pain may seem like a complicated endeavor, it can be simplified by following a few steps. The history and physical are always important because they allow differentiation between the 3 categories of back pain. For nonspecific back pain, start with self-care and stretching, and, if need be, expand treatment to include pharmacologic and nonpharmacologic therapies. Patients who do not respond to these treatments should be considered for interdisciplinary rehabilitation.

REFERENCES

1. Available at: http://www.chirobase.org/07Strategy/AHCPR/ahcprclinician.html. Accessed March 18, 2012.
2. Chou R, Qaseem A, Snow V, et al. Diagnosis and treatment of low back pain: a joint clinical practice guideline from the American College of Physicians and the American Pain Society. Ann Intern Med 2007;147:478–91.
3. Pengel LH, Herbert RD, Maher CG, et al. Acute low back pain: systematic review of its prognosis. BMJ 2003;327:323.
4. Chou R, Huffman L. Evaluation and management of low back pain: evidence review. American Pain Society, in press.

The Physiology of Low Back Pain

Lenny Salzberg, MD

KEYWORDS

• Pain • Low back • Intervertebral disc • Anatomy • Physiology

KEY POINTS

- Pain by definition is subjective. A variety of neural pathways are involved in the generation and propagation of pain.
- Pain is emotional. Pain pathways interact with the limbic system; this interaction modulates pain. The experience of pain is related to the experience of past pain.
- Many potential pain generators are present in the low back. The most likely source of pain is the intervertebral disc. Treating pain requires a multifactorial approach, because pain is complex.

PAIN DEFINED

What is pain? As Supreme Court Justice Potter Stewart famously said in 1964 when describing pornography, "I know it when I see it." Subjective experiences are difficult to categorize. According to the International Association for the Study of Pain (IASP),[1] pain is an unpleasant sensory and emotional experience associated with actual or potential tissue damage. Based on this description, a few things become apparent: pain is by definition subjective; pain has an emotional component; and pain may or may not be caused by any actual damage. How does this relate to the approach to patients with low back pain? When physicians try to understand a patient's subjective experience of pain, they need to address the emotional component of pain first and foremost, and only then try to understand what the actual or potential tissue damage was that caused the pain. Understanding the spinal cord mechanisms of pain and knowing the pain generators in the back may help illuminate why some of the treatments used for back pain are effective.

Back pain is common; it is the fifth most common reason for all physician visits in the United States.[2] Approximately half of adults have low back pain during any given year, and approximately two-thirds of the population has low back pain at some time in their lives.[3] The pathophysiology of pain is still not completely understood, but some knowledge exists of what structures can be pain generators and how pain is transmitted. The anatomy and physiology of the low back are complex. Whether pain is generated from problems with the intervertebral discs, facet joint arthritis, vertebral

Family Medicine Residency, Duke/Southern Regional AHEC, 1601 Owen Drive, Fayetteville, NC 28304, USA
E-mail address: lenny.salzberg@sr-ahec.org

Prim Care Clin Office Pract 39 (2012) 487–498
http://dx.doi.org/10.1016/j.pop.2012.06.014 **primarycare.theclinics.com**
0095-4543/12/$ – see front matter © 2012 Elsevier Inc. All rights reserved.

misalignment, muscles, ligaments, fascia, or neural structures is difficult to determine. To complicate matters, the cognitive behavioral components of the perception of pain, discussed elsewhere in this issue by Garland and colleagues, often confuse diagnosis, management, and long-term prognosis of patients with low back pain. Occam's razor states that the simplest explanation that fits all the facts is probably correct. How can Occam's razor be applied to the question of what causes low back pain? Unfortunately, there is not one simple explanation that fits all the facts; a multitude of potential pain generators exist. Prevention of injury and treatment of pain all rely on current knowledge of neuronal pathways and neurogenic mediators. Knowledge of this final common pathway can help guide diagnostic and treatment guidelines.

PAIN TRANSMISSION

Independent of the pain generator, sensory impulses from the low back are conducted through myelinated A beta fibers, thinly myelinated A delta fibers, and unmyelinated C fibers to the dorsal root ganglia (DRG) (**Fig. 1**).[4] The thick A beta fibers transmit information about light touch, not pain, quickly and with a low activation threshold. Less myelinated A delta fibers and C fibers transmit pain, do so much more slowly, and have a much higher activation threshold.

Substance P, calcitonin gene-related peptide (CGRP), and vasoactive intestinal polypeptide (VIP) are peptides that are released by peripheral and central neurons to transmit pain in response to inflammation or injury. In addition to transmitting pain, these neuropeptides may be involved in inflammation,[5] and may work synergistically with each other. Inflammation can trigger pain transmission in other sites.

The DRG are sometimes referred to as the brain of the spinal segment, and are thought to be instrumental in modulating pain.[5,6] Proximity to the DRG may be related to pain severity; the closer the anatomic disruption is to the DRG, the greater the pain.

Sensory nerves terminate in the dorsal horn of the spinal cord.[4] The dorsal horn has laminae, or layers. The more superficial layers (I and II) are where most pain fibers terminate (although some do reach deeper). In these superficial layers are cells that respond to the neurotransmitters (eg, substance P, CGRP, VIP) released by A delta and C fibers. The deeper layers (III–VI) are where most tactile (A beta) fibers terminate. Within the spinal cord itself, cells are present that connect the layers. Within a deeper layer (lamina V) of the dorsal horn nucleus are cells that receive input from all three types of neurons. These cells, known as wide dynamic range neurons (WDR), can then transmit impulses in a graded fashion depending on stimulus intensity. They also can experience the "wind-up" phenomenon: if they are repetitively stimulated, they will have an increased response with each stimulus.

Pain that was transmitted to the dorsal horn from the low back is then transmitted to the brain.[4] Fibers from the two superficial laminae travel to the parabrachial area (PB) and the periaqueductal gray (PAG) area, where they are affected by the limbic system. The limbic system colors the painful experience with emotion. Impulses are then fed down from the brainstem back to the dorsal horn, modulating spinal processing of pain. Fibers from the deeper lamina (V) project mainly to the thalamus via the spinothalamic tract. Once the impulses are in the thalamus, individuals become conscious of pain. From the thalamus, the pain impulse goes to the cerebral cortex, where location and intensity are perceived in the postcentral gyrus. The frontal lobes help give the pain emotional context, whereas the temporal lobe provides memories of pain.

Descending neurons of the spinal cord and midbrain can inhibit pain transmission. The brain transmits gate-blocking impulses through the brain stem and spinal cord to provide pain relief. Endorphins are released in the dorsal horn to diminish pain.

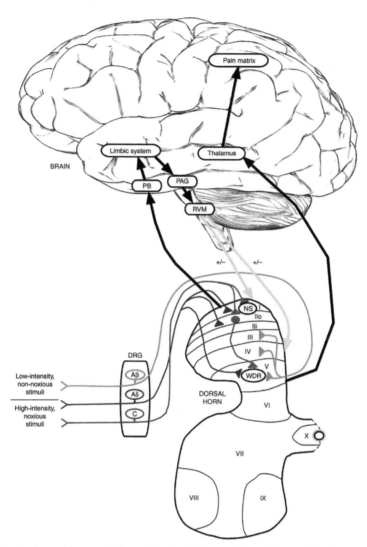

Fig. 1. Pain pathways from periphery to brain. Primary afferent fibers (Aβ, Aδ, and C fibers) transmit impulses from the periphery, through the dorsal root ganglion (DRG), and into the dorsal horn of the spinal cord. Nociceptive specific (NS) cells are mainly found in the superficial dorsal horn (laminae I–II), whereas most wide dynamic ranges (WDRs) are located deeper (lamina V). Projection neurones from lamina I innervate areas, such as the parabrachial area (PB) and periaqueductal gray (PAG), and these pathways are affected by limbic areas. From here, descending pathways (*yellow arrows*) from brainstem nuclei, such as the rostral ventromedial medulla (RVM), are activated and modulate spinal processing. Lamina V neurones mainly project to the thalamus (spinothalamic tract), and from here the various cortical regions forming the pain matrix (primary and secondary somatosensory, insular, anterior cingulate, and prefrontal cortices) are activated. (*From* D'Mello R, Dickenson AH. Spinal cord mechanisms of pain. Br J Anaesth 2008;101(1):9; with permission.)

Some cells in the dorsal horn of the spinal cord learn to respond to signals other than painful signals in anticipation of pain. They act like a switch stuck in the on position, amplifying the pain signal up to the thalamus. They can exaggerate or create pain. Sometimes the central modulation of pain can also be dysfunctional; it does not blunt the pain as it should. These features help explain the wide variation in pain perception and the development of chronic pain. In chronic pain, normally innocuous stimuli may generate a pain response.

Within the spinal cord are a variety of neurotransmitters and receptors. Glutamate is essential for pain signaling at every level.[4] α-Amino-3-hydroxy-5-methyl-4-isoxazolepropionic acid receptors and N-methyl-D-aspartate receptors are present and play an important role, such as in relation to magnesium plugs, calcium channels, and sodium channels. Serotonin plays a role in modulating pain with spinal serotonin receptors present. Each of these are areas in which medications and complementary techniques may have an effect.

ANATOMIC CAUSES

Where is the pain coming from? When trying to locate the anatomic cause of low back pain, an important question is, "Does the back pain originate in the back?" Low back pain can be caused by problems outside the back, including neoplasms, pancreatitis, nephrolithiasis, aortic aneurysm, endocarditis, and viral syndromes. Nonmechanical or systemic causes of acute low back pain are uncommon in the family medicine setting (≤3%).[7] As good family physicians know, these potential causes should be eliminated through taking a good history and performing a thorough physical examination before concentrating on the spine.

The spine is best understood anatomically as an integrated, interdependent, dynamic biologic structure,[8] rather than as independent units. To understand the interplay of the structures, however, one must first know what they are. What elements are "the back"? The intervertebral disc, the zygapophyseal (facet) joints, the sacroiliac joint, ligaments of the back, muscle, and fascia are all potential sources of pain in the low back. These "pain generators" have varied innervation, which contributes to the complexity of understanding and localizing low back pain.

THE INTERVERTEBRAL DISC

The basic units of low back anatomy, and one on which most attention must be focused, is the intervertebral disc. This disc is a complex cushion between vertebrae. It absorbs the loads of the spinal column and dissipates these loads to allow smooth movement of the spine.[9] The disc has a unique structure (**Fig. 2**). It has an inner gelatinous portion, the nucleus pulposis, surrounded by a firm outer layer, the annulus fibrosis. One way to envision this is to picture a stress ball, frequently used in physical therapy; these consist of gel inside a rubber or cloth skin. When you squeeze a stress ball, the ball deforms, absorbing the force. It then returns to its original shape after it is destressed. The difference between a stress ball and a disc, however, is that the intervertebral disc is alive and has active components to its function.

The gelatinous portion of the intervertebral disc, the nucleus pulposis, is made of an extracellular matrix of type II collagen, proteoglycans, and other proteins made by chondrocytes, forming a gelatinous core.[8] The proteoglycans link together, giving the nucleus pulposis hydrostatic properties. Normally the nucleus pulposis is 70% to 80% water.[9] It has both hydraulic and ion transport properties, allowing for compression and decompression. The gelatinous property of the nucleus pulposis helps the disc maintain structural integrity through the variety of movements the spine undergoes: flexion, extension,

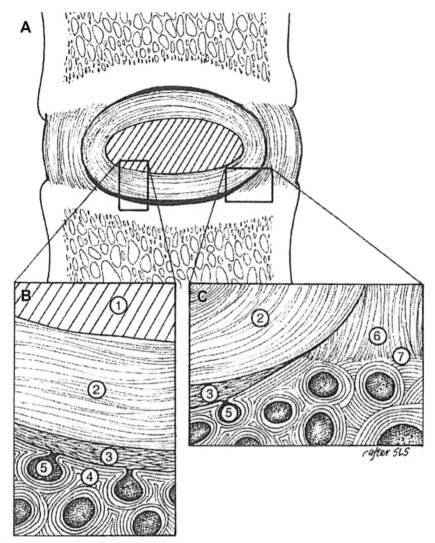

Fig. 2. The intervertebral disc. (*A*) Fibers are arranged in a lamellar fashion. (*B*) and (*C*) Magnified view of disc. 1. nucleus pulposis; 2. annulus fibrosis; 3. cartilagenous end plate; 4. bony end plate; 5. vascular channel. (*Adapted from* Dupuis PR. The anatomy of the lumbosacral spine. In: Kirkaldy-Willis WH, Burton CV, editors. Managing low back pain. 3rd edition. New York: Churchill Livingstone; 1992. p. 10–27; with permission.)

and rotation. The nucleus pulposis is mostly acellular. Only 1% to 5% of the intervertebral disc tissue volume is made up of cells, and these are predominantly in the annulus.[9] Like bone tissue with a dynamic balance of osteoblasts making bone and osteoclasts destroying bone, in a healthy disc the extracellular matrix is in a state of flux: it is continuously produced and broken down. Synthesis is activated by growth factors (fibroblast growth factor, transforming growth factor, and insulin-like growth factor), whereas destruction is mediated by interleukin 1, interferon, and tumor necrosis factor alpha.[8] The nucleus pulposis is avascular. Nutrition diffuses through the inner annulus fibers to the matrix. The nucleus pulposis in a normal disc has no innervation.

The "rubber or cloth skin" of the intervertebral disc is the annulus fibrosis. This outer skin must have high tensile strength to deal with all of the forces applied to it. The annulus fibrosis is made of sheets of interlacing type I collagen, synthesized by chondrocytes (see **Fig. 2**). This collagen network, in addition to providing tensile strength, limits the expansion of the nucleus pulposis, allowing the disc to deform and return to its original shape. In a healthy disc, blood vessels are limited to the outer rings of the annulus fibrosis. Innervation of the intervertebral disc only reaches the outer posterior aspect of the annulus fibrosis; innervation deep to the outer annulus is not seen in healthy discs.[8] In damaged discs, innervations through the annulus fibrosis into the nucleus pulposis occur. Between the vertebral bone and the intervertebral disc are the cartilaginous end plates. These sheets of hyaline cartilage have pores for diffusion of nutrition for the disc.

Are abnormal discs the pain generators causing acute or chronic low back pain? Intervertebral disc herniation has been described since Dandy[10] in 1929 as the possible source of low back pain. In Dandy's case study, two patients experienced sudden onset of severe low back pain and had presumed tumors of the cauda equina. Disc herniation was found unexpectedly in the operating room. By 1934, disc disease was more widely accepted as the cause of low back pain, as described by Mixter and Barr[11] in the *New England Journal of Medicine*.

Pathologic intervertebral disc degeneration without herniation is also linked to back pain.[12] When a disc is damaged, the tenuous balance of anabolic and catabolic activity is shifted toward catabolism. The number of chondrocytes in the matrix and in the annulus fibrosis decrease, and collagen fiber types in the nucleus pulposis change from type II to type I, causing the nucleus pulposis to become less spongy and more fibrotic. Because fewer proteoglycans are present, the disc becomes less hydrostatic and desiccates. Degenerated discs, as opposed to healthy discs, which have no innervation of the nucleus pulposis or the inner annulus, develop pathologic innervation with pain fibers into both the inner annulus and the nucleus pulposis. These pain fibers in the disc itself may be the pain generators for low back pain.

Up to 90% of people by the age of 50 years will develop degenerative disc changes.[13] The relationship between intervertebral disc degeneration and low back pain may be from a variety of factors other than pain in the disc itself. Local chemical mediation of pain may be produced by cytokines released as the nucleus pulposis degrades. Both nitrous oxide and phospholipase A2 have been implicated in animal studies[14,15] as causes of hyperalgesia. Extrusion of nucleus pulposis into the epidural space evokes an autoimmune response,[16–18] which activates a cascade of destruction: inflammatory cells secrete cytokines, macrophages are recruited, and proteinases are released that weaken the posterior longitudinal ligament. A proliferation of vessels and sensory nerves occurs at the end plate adjacent to the degenerated disc. These nerves at the end plate may be the pain generator when a disc degenerates.

OTHER PAIN GENERATORS

Is disc degeneration caused by mechanical factors? Discs can withstand a wide range of forces. The vertebral end plate seems to be more vulnerable to excessive load than the intervertebral disc.[8] Conditions that reduce blood flow to the spine are associated with disc damage, and smoking can cause increased disc herniation (yet another reason patients should be counseled to quit smoking).[19,20]

What evidence exists that the intervertebral disc is the main pain generator of low back pain? The most reliable test of the intervertebral disc as a pain generator is provocation discography[12,21] (evidence level A: meta-analysis). This diagnostic test involves placing a needle into the disc under fluoroscopy followed by contrast insertion. The contrast distends the disc, reproducing the pain. In one study, the prevalence of discogenic low back pain was 39%.[22]

Is disc disease the sole answer? MRI findings of abnormal discs are similar to right upper quadrant ultrasound findings of stones in the gall bladder: they do not always correlate with pain.[23] What are other possible causes of pain? Could the disc degeneration cause sequelae outside of the disc itself, which cause pain? Can low back pain be independent of disc degeneration?

Desiccated fibrotic discs alter the alignment of the spinal column, including facet joints, ligaments, and muscles. Are these alternate sources of low back pain?

The intervertebral discs separate the vertebrae anteriorly. Posteriorly, the spinal segments articulate with each other at joints, known as zygapophyseal joints or, more commonly, facet joints. These zygapophyses stick out of the end of a vertebra to lock on the next vertebra, making the backbone more stable. As is the case with other synovial joints, these joints can become inflamed and show degenerative changes. Similar to osteoarthritis in the knee causing pain, it makes sense that osteoarthritis of the zygapophyseal joints could be a pain generator.

Each lumbar spinal segment has two joints. They are formed by a right inferior articular facet of one vertebra articulating with the right superior articular facet of the vertebra below (**Fig. 3**), and a left inferior articular facet articulating with the left superior facet of the vertebra below. The articular facets vary in shape and orientation at different lumbar levels, providing more or less surface area in contact. These factors vary the patterns of resistance the joints provide. Lower lumbar level joints have more surface area in contact, resisting forward displacement, whereas higher lumbar level joints have a different orientation and allow forward displacement, but resist rotation. Like other joints elsewhere in the body, these joints have hyaline cartilage and a synovial membrane surrounded by a joint capsule. The capsule contains 1.0 to 1.5 mL of fluid.[8] The zygapophyseal joint is richly innervated by nerves from two branches

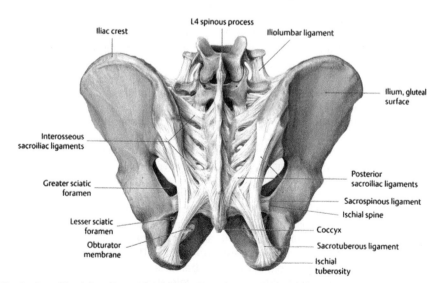

Fig. 3. Sacroiliac joint. (*From* Vleeming A, Stoeckart R. The role of the pelvic girdle in coupling the spine and legs; a clinical-anatomic perspective on pelvic stability. In: Vleeming A, Mooney V, Stoeckart R, editors. Movement, stability and lumbopelvic pain: integration of research and therapy. London: Elsevier; 2007. p. 115; with permission.)

from consecutive vertebral levels. These same branches also innervate the multifidus muscle, the interspinous ligament, and the periosteum of the neural arch.[8] Innervation may also come from the dorsal root ganglion (DRG) and the paravertebral sympathetic ganglion. An estimated 15% to 40%[24] of lumbar pain is caused by zygapophyseal joint pain.

Another joint in the low back is the sacroiliac joint. The sacrum is the large, triangular wedge-shaped bone that together with the two iliac bones form the posterior wall of the pelvis. The superior portion of the joint is more like a symphysis, whereas the inferior portion is more like a synovial joint. The sacroiliac joint is supported by multiple ligaments, which maintain its shape and position (see **Fig. 3**). Ligaments support it to prevent rocking or rotation. The joint works to absorb mechanical force from the legs across the pelvic girdle. Usually the joint itself does not have much movement. The sacroiliac joint is essential to a variety of pelvic movements during standing and walking, and is involved in core stability.

The sacroiliac joint is also known to be a cause of low back pain. Mechanical changes, inflammation, and trauma all occur in the sacroiliac joint. Osteoarthritis affects this joint, and repetitive strain also can contribute to pain. A unique cause of sacroiliac pain is pregnancy. Pregnancy contributes to sacroiliac pain through weight gain, lordosis, and ligamentous laxity.

In addition to discs and joints, ligaments are also present in the back. These include the ligamentum flavum, longitudinal ligaments, interspinous and supraspinous ligaments, and iliolumbar ligament. The ligamentum flavum is more elastic (80% elastic fibers, 20% collagenous fibers) than other ligaments. Its role is to prevent buckling of the vertebral column during flexion and extension. When disc herniation occurs, the ligamentum flavum itself buckles, which may contribute to nerve root compression.[25] In patients with spinal stenosis, calcification and thickening of the mostly elastic ligamentum flavum is commonly seen.

There are both anterior and posterior longitudinal ligaments. Their role is to resist separation of the intervertebral discs during extension and flexion, respectively. These longitudinal ligaments cover the entire vertebral column. Interspinous ligaments connect consecutive spinous processes. They serve as an anchor, together with the thoracolumbar fascia and multifidus sheath, providing central support to the spine.[8] The interspinous ligament can be a source of referred pain to the spine, trunk, abdomen, and limbs. The iliolumbar ligament provides a strong attachment for L5 and the ilium and restrains lumbosacral movement, including side bending, flexion, and extension, and its primary role may be proprioceptive.

Moving all of these structures are the muscles of the lumbosacral spine, including the multifidus, interspinales/intertransversalis, and erector spinae. Other muscles are also important for back health, although they do not directly move the spine, including the transversus abdominis, psoas major, gluteus maximus, and piriformis muscles.

The multifidus muscle has short and long fibers. The short fibers connect two adjacent vertebrae, originating on the vertebra above and inserting more laterally on the vertebra below. The long fibers are sets of five fascicles, attaching a vertebra to multiple vertebrae below, and to the iliac crest and the sacrum. These muscles are active during standing, sitting, walking, trunk movement, and lifting. They facilitate a self-bracing mechanism through compressing the intervertebral discs. They counteract the abdominal muscles during lumbar flexion, facilitate lumbar lordosis, and transfer energy from the upper body to the lower extremities. The interspinales and intertransversalis muscles connect consecutive spinal processes (**Fig. 4**). They are primarily proprioceptive. The erector spinae muscles form an aponeurosis that connects the lumbar spine and the ilium. They counteract lumbar flexion and derotate the spine.

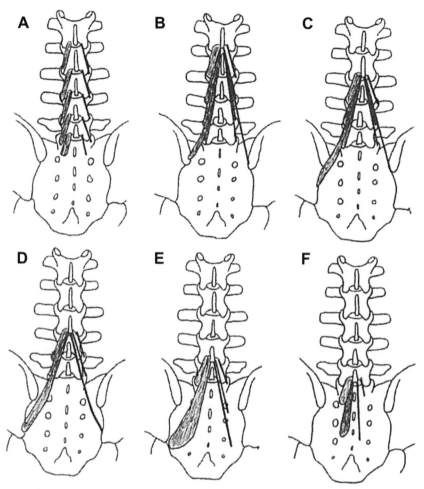

Fig. 4. Multifidus muscle anatomy. (*From* Bogduk N. The lumbar muscles and their fascia. In: Bogduk N, editor. Clinical anatomy of the lumbar spine. 4th edition. London: Elsevier; 2005. p. 102; with permission.)

Fascia, a multilayered soft tissue sheath that divides muscles, provides a continuum throughout the back uniting and integrating the muscles, ligaments, and tendons in the region. The posterior layer of the thoracolumbar fascia transfers force between the spine and the extremities. Fascia, an integral component of the anatomy of the low back, also may be a pain generator.

MANAGEMENT

Does establishing a specific anatomic diagnosis of low back pain change the management of the pain? According to the 2007 American College of Physicians (ACP)/American Pain Society (APS) guidelines for diagnosis and treatment of low back pain, the answer is no. In these guidelines,[26] the first recommendation is to conduct a focused history and physical examination to help place patients with low back pain into one of three broad categories: nonspecific low back pain, back pain associated with radiculopathy or spinal stenosis, or back pain potentially associated with another specific spinal cause. The history should include assessment of psychosocial risk factors, which predict risk for chronic disabling back pain. According to the guidelines, labeling most patients with low back pain using specific anatomic diagnoses does not improve outcomes (evidence level C: expert opinion).[26]

Despite this recommendation, treatments may be developed in the future that target a specific pain generator. Understanding what the pain generators could be will help explain why different treatment options may be effective. Furthermore, understanding the cause of low back pain may help physicians prevent low back pain in patients in whom it has not yet developed. Finally, understanding what causes low back pain will allow physicians to provide information to patients when the pain can no longer be fixed.

Understanding the possible generators and the neuroanatomy of pain helps better explain how medications that currently are used for pain may work. Systemic antiinflammatory medications may shut down the inflammatory cascade that ensues after substance P, CGRP, and other neuropeptides are released. Topical antiinflammatory drugs may similarly work at the site of the DRG. Medications such as lidocaine patches work on the sodium channels in pain transmission. They may "shut the gate" through which sensations other than pain are aberrantly transmitting ascending pain. Opiates work on the descending pain pathways, modulating pain in a similar fashion to local endorphins.

Complementary and alternative techniques, such as acupuncture and chiropractic manipulation, probably work at the level of the DRG, blocking the release of the pain cascade, and at the dorsal horn, modulating and inhibiting pain. Chiropractic manipulation may also work through realigning structures that are displaced by the mechanical change in a disc as it loses its structure. Spinal manipulative therapy (SMT) distracts the facet joints[27] and forcefully stretches the paraspinal muscles. It may be that SMT disrupts the pain-spasm-pain cycle, but this mechanism is not proven.[27] One explanation of the effects of SMT may be that it alters central sensory processing by removing mechanical or chemical stimuli from paraspinous tissues.[28] Removing these stimuli may reduce the "wind-up" phenomena. SMT may have some effect on the interplay of tactile stimuli and painful stimuli in lamina V of the Dorsal Horn.

Acupuncture analgesia stimulates the release of ß-endorphin, enkephalin, endomorphin, and dynorphin,[29] which modulate pain. It may also release serotonin, which also works via the descending inhibitory pathway.[30] Brain regions affected by acupuncture include the nucleus raphe magnus, periaqueductal gray, locus coeruleus, arcuate nucleus, preoptic area, nucleus submedius, habenular nucleus, accumbens nucleus, caudate nucleus, septal area, and amygdala.[31]

SUMMARY

Pain by definition is subjective. A variety of neural pathways are involved in the generation and propagation of pain. Pain is emotional. Pain pathways interact with the limbic system, and this interaction modulates pain. The experience of pain is related to the experience of past pain. Many potential pain generators are present in the low back. The most likely source of pain is the intervertebral disc. Treating pain requires a multifactorial approach, because pain is very complex.

REFERENCES

1. IASP taxonomy. International Association for the Study of Pain Web site. Available at: http://www.iasp-pain.org/Content/NavigationMenu/GeneralResourceLinks/Pain Definitions/default.htm. Accessed February 8, 2012.

2. Hart LG, Deyo RA, Cherkin DC. Physician office visits for low back pain. frequency, clinical evaluation, and treatment patterns from a U.S. national survey. Spine (Phila Pa 1976) 1995;20(1):11–9.
3. Deyo RA, Mirza SK, Martin BI. Back pain prevalence and visit rates: estimates from U.S. national surveys, 2002. Spine (Phila Pa 1976) 2006;31(23):2724–7.
4. D'Mello R, Dickenson AH. Spinal cord mechanisms of pain. Br J Anaesth 2008; 101(1):8–16.
5. Weinstein J. Neurogenic and nonneurogenic pain and inflammatory mediators. Orthop Clin North Am 1991;22(2):235–46.
6. Harrington JF, Messier AA, Bereiter D, et al. Herniated lumbar disc material as a source of free glutamate available to affect pain signals through the dorsal root ganglion. Spine (Phila Pa 1976) 2000;25(8):929–36.
7. Elder N, Smucker D. Back and neck pain. 322nd edition. Leawood (KS): American Academy of Family Physicians; 2006.
8. Vora AJ, Doerr KD, Wolfer LR. Functional anatomy and pathophysiology of axial low back pain: disc, posterior elements, sacroiliac joint, and associated pain generators. Phys Med Rehabil Clin N Am 2010;21(4):679–709.
9. Biyani A, Andersson GB. Low back pain: pathophysiology and management. J Am Acad Orthop Surg 2004;12(2):106–15.
10. Dandy WE. Loose cartilage from intervertebral disk simulating tumor of the spinal cord. Arch Surg 1929;19(4):660–72.
11. Mixter WJ, Barr JS. Rupture of the intervertebral disc with involvement of the spinal canal. N Engl J Med 1934;211:210–5.
12. Schwarzer AC, Aprill CN, Derby R, et al. The prevalence and clinical features of internal disc disruption in patients with chronic low back pain. Spine (Phila Pa 1976) 1995;20(17):1878–83.
13. Miller JA, Schmatz C, Schultz AB. Lumbar disc degeneration: correlation with age, sex, and spine level in 600 autopsy specimens. Spine (Phila Pa 1976) 1988;13(2):173–8.
14. Kawakami M, Tamaki T, Hayashi N, et al. Possible mechanism of painful radiculopathy in lumbar disc herniation. Clin Orthop Relat Res 1998;(351):241–51.
15. Saal JS, Franson RC, Dobrow R, et al. High levels of inflammatory phospholipase A2 activity in lumbar disc herniations. Spine (Phila Pa 1976) 1990;15(7): 674–8.
16. Nemoto O, Yamagishi M, Yamada H, et al. Matrix metalloproteinase-3 production by human degenerated intervertebral disc. J Spinal Disord 1997;10(6):493–8.
17. Liu J, Roughley PJ, Mort JS. Identification of human intervertebral disc stromelysin and its involvement in matrix degradation. J Orthop Res 1991;9(4):568–75.
18. Doita M, Kanatani T, Ozaki T, et al. Influence of macrophage infiltration of herniated disc tissue on the production of matrix metalloproteinases leading to disc resorption. Spine (Phila Pa 1976) 2001;26(14):1522–7.
19. Kauppila LI. Can low-back pain be due to lumbar-artery disease? Lancet 1995; 346(8979):888–9.
20. Kauppila LI, Penttila A, Karhunen PJ, et al. Lumbar disc degeneration and atherosclerosis of the abdominal aorta. Spine (Phila Pa 1976) 1994;19(8):923–9.
21. Wolfer LR, Derby R, Lee JE, et al. Systematic review of lumbar provocation discography in asymptomatic subjects with a meta-analysis of false-positive rates. Pain Physician 2008;11(4):513–38.
22. Manchikanti L, Singh V, Rivera JJ, et al. Effectiveness of caudal epidural injections in discogram positive and negative chronic low back pain. Pain Physician 2002;5(1):18–29.

23. Delamarter RB, Howard MW, Goldstein T, et al. Percutaneous lumbar discectomy. preoperative and postoperative magnetic resonance imaging. J Bone Joint Surg Am 1995;77(4):578–84.

24. Sehgal N, Shah RV, McKenzie-Brown AM, et al. Diagnostic utility of facet (zygapophysial) joint injections in chronic spinal pain: a systematic review of evidence. Pain Physician 2005;8(2):211–24.

25. Okuda T, Fujimoto Y, Tanaka N, et al. Morphological changes of the ligamentum flavum as a cause of nerve root compression. Eur Spine J 2005;14(3):277–86.

26. Chou R, Qaseem A, Snow V, et al. Diagnosis and treatment of low back pain: a joint clinical practice guideline from the American College of Physicians and the American Pain Society. Ann Intern Med 2007;147(7):478–91.

27. Maigne JY, Vautravers P. Mechanism of action of spinal manipulative therapy. Joint Bone Spine 2003;70(5):336–41.

28. Pickar JG. Neurophysiological effects of spinal manipulation. Spine J 2002;2(5):357–71.

29. Han JS. Acupuncture and endorphins. Neurosci Lett 2004;361(1–3):258–61.

30. Lin JG, Chen WL. Acupuncture analgesia: a review of its mechanisms of actions. Am J Chin Med 2008;36(4):635–45.

31. Zhao ZQ. Neural mechanism underlying acupuncture analgesia. Prog Neurobiol 2008;85(4):355–75.

Low Back Pain: Pharmacologic Management

Susan M. Miller, PharmD, MBA, BCPS, FCCP[a,b,*]

KEYWORDS

- Low back pain • Pharmacologic treatment • Opioid therapy
- Evidence-based practice

KEY POINTS

- Treatment for low back pain involves a balance between patient expectations for pain relief and the possible pain relief that pharmacologic treatment can provide.
- Education regarding medications, goals for treatment, and expected outcomes should occur early and often with patients during the course of treatment for low back pain.
- Acetaminophen or NSAIDs are first line treatments for low back pain.
- Opioids should be reserved as a last choice medication for low back pain treatment due to lack of evidence and potential for abuse.
- Although strong evidence is lacking, other possible treatments for low back pain include muscle relaxants, antidepressants, antipsychotics, and antiseizure medications.

INTRODUCTION

Low back pain is a prevalent complaint among Americans, with approximately 7.6 million people (16.8% of the population) complaining of back pain in 2005.[1] A 2009 report from the Centers for Disease Control and Prevention articulates that back pain falls only behind arthritis/rheumatism as a reason for disability in the United States.[1] It is the leading cause of disability for adults younger than 45 years and sufferers lose almost a full day of work (5.2 hours) each week due to low back pain.[2] This situation translates to a loss of more than $100 billion in productivity for the United States workforce.[3]

Most people with low back pain visit their primary care physician for treatment. Adequate treatment of low back pain is essential, but has been challenging for many primary care physicians. During a short office visit for low back pain the provider must determine the acuity of the pain, whether it is acute or chronic, the validity of the complaint, and the best treatment options. Often, the provider has to deal with

The author has nothing to disclose.
[a] Duke/Southern Regional Area Health Education Family Medicine Residency Program, Fayetteville, NC, USA; [b] University of North Carolina Chapel Hill Eshelman School of Pharmacy, NC, USA
* Cape Fear Valley/Southern Regional Area Health Education Center, 1601 Owen Drive, Fayetteville, NC 28305.
E-mail address: susan.miller@sr-ahec.org

Prim Care Clin Office Pract 39 (2012) 499–510
http://dx.doi.org/10.1016/j.pop.2012.06.005   **primarycare.theclinics.com**
0095-4543/12/$ – see front matter © 2012 Elsevier Inc. All rights reserved.

completion of disability paperwork. For the most part, primary care physicians are not sufficiently trained to treat low back pain as a chronic illness. Most patients with low back pain can be treated in the primary care environment, provided the physician has enough knowledge of the medications used to treat low back pain.[3]

Acute low back pain is defined as that which will resolve over time and lasts no longer than 6 weeks.[4] The main treatment goal for acute low back pain is to control the pain and maintain function, allowing symptoms to diminish on their own. Many (50%–75%) patients have spontaneous resolution at 4 weeks, and upward of 90% have full resolution at 6 weeks.[5] In comparison, chronic low back pain lasts longer than 3 months and is more difficult to treat. Patients with chronic back pain tend to have exacerbations that can recur over time. Unfortunately, patients with chronic low back pain may not obtain complete resolution of their pain. For these patients, the goal is continual pain management and prevention of future exacerbations.[6] For patients with chronic low back pain, the ultimate functional outcomes often depend more on psychosocial factors than on medical treatment.[6]

When low back pain first occurs, the treatment goal should initially be to achieve a total cure for the back pain, but as time progresses the goal may shift toward pain reduction and maintenance of function. Patient education is essential in regards to expected treatment outcomes, as patients often have unrealistic expectations regarding pain relief and functioning capabilities.[4] Often there is a large gap between the patient's expectations and what the treatment plan can offer. Establishing goals and expectations with interim assessments toward goal achievement can be helpful.[7]

TREATMENT GUIDELINES

The most recent guidelines for the treatment of low back pain were published jointly by the American College of Physicians and the American Pain Society in 2007.[8] Of the 7 recommendations listed, one recommendation focuses on the use of medications for treatment of low back pain. This recommendation supports the use of those medications with proven benefits, combined with self-care and education, to treat patients with low back pain. The main consensus is that the majority of patients can be treated with acetaminophen or nonsteroidal anti-inflammatory drugs (NSAIDs).

Since the publication of this guideline, the American Pain Society and the American Academy of Pain Medicine has published a clinical guideline on the use of chronic opioid therapy for noncancer pain (**Box 1**).[9] Their definition of noncancer pain includes back pain. The guideline contains 14 recommendations regarding the long-term use of opioids, to include such areas as initiating and titrating opioid therapy, methadone use, monitoring opioid use, opioid side effects, and opioid management plans. Primary care physicians may find this guideline helpful if it is necessary to prescribe opioids in the treatment of low back pain.

GENERAL TREATMENT PRINCIPLES FOR LOW BACK PAIN

In general, the treatment of acute and chronic low back pain involves a balance between patient expectations for pain relief and the amount of pain relief that medications can provide.[7] Early patient education regarding what can be expected from pharmacotherapy will lead to more realistic expectations for the patient. Psychosocial factors and emotional distress are stronger predictors of outcomes of low back pain than either physical examination findings or severity and duration of pain. Physicians should assess patients for depression, unemployment, job dissatisfaction, somatization disorder, and psychological distress, as these conditions tend to delay recovery.[6]

Box 1
American Pain Society and American Academy of Pain Medicine treatment guidelines for noncancer pain recommendations for clinicians

1. Select patient for chronic opioid use using risk stratification

2. Communicate risks and benefits of chronic opioid use and potential use of pain management plan for documentation with patient

3. Consider initial use of opioid therapy on a trial basis, with individualized drug choice, initial dosing and titration

4. Use caution if methadone is selected, and use caution during initiation and titration by clinicians familiar with its unique properties

5. Perform monitoring for efficacy, adverse effects, and possible diversion

6. Frequent monitoring and possible consultation with behavioral health specialist for patients with history of drug abuse or psychiatric issues

7. Reassess for benefits and risks of opioid use and consider opioid rotation if patient receiving inadequate efficacy or intolerable adverse effects while attempting to escalate opioid dosage

8. Anticipate and treat opioid-related adverse effects

9. Integrate psychotherapeutic interventions, interdisciplinary therapy, and adjunctive nonopioid therapies

10. Counsel patients on potential for cognitive impairment that may affect daily activities (ie, driving)

11. Help patients identify a medical home responsible for their overall care

12. Consider as needed opioids for breakthrough pain if opioids are prescribed around the clock

13. Counsel female patients about the benefits and risks of chronic opioid therapy during pregnancy and after delivery

14. Familiarize themselves with state and federal regulations regarding opioid prescribing

---

When deciding to prescribe medications for the treatment of low back pain, the clinician should weigh the benefits against the risks of the medications as they relate to the specific patient to be treated. By and large, medication use for low back pain should be for the shortest time possible and discontinued when there appears to be no more benefit to its use.[8,9] Extended courses of medications should only be used if the patient clearly exhibits continued benefits from therapy without major adverse effects. Throughout the treatment period, documentation of patient's pain relief and quality of life subsequent to prescribed therapies is crucial. Pain scores should be documented in the patient's record as the fifth vital sign, using a visual analog scale, or on a scale of 1 up to a maximum of 10.

Published guidelines for the treatment of low back pain recommend that clinicians select medications with documented efficacy data and use these in combination with education and self-care in the treatment plan for a patient with low back pain.[8,9] Before prescribing any medications for low back pain, the guidelines recommend that clinicians complete a variety of patient assessments, to include pain and functional deficits and a benefits/risk analysis of the medications, in an attempt to select the best care for the patient.[8,9] In addition, costs of medications must be considered as part of the treatment plan.

At best, the medications used to treat low back pain have been shown to be moderately effective for short-term treatment of acute back pain. With medication, thankfully most patients (90%) recover within a couple of weeks of the onset of low back pain.[6,10] For some patients it can take up to 2 months or more for recovery to occur.[6] Unfortunately, some patients continue to have intermittent or chronic low back pain for 6 months or more.[10] Social, clinical, and economic factors may help predict which patients may transition from acute to chronic low back pain.[7,10]

MEDICATIONS FOR THE TREATMENT OF LOW BACK PAIN
Acetaminophen

Acetaminophen has not been studied specifically for the treatment of low back pain. An ongoing Australian trial, in the recruitment phase as of late 2011, will be the first randomized, placebo-controlled trial assessing whether 4000 mg of acetaminophen leads to a more rapid recovery from acute low back pain in comparison with placebo.[11] Even without evidence to support its use, many consider acetaminophen to be the drug of choice to alleviate low back pain.[5–8] Acetaminophen is a reasonable choice, because of its more favorable safety profile and low cost compared with other treatment options.

In 2011, the Food and Drug Administration (FDA) dictated limits regarding the maximum tablet strength (325 mg) for prescription acetaminophen-containing products (ie, Vicodin, Lortab, and so forth).[12] The limit on tablet strength allows providers to continue to prescribe 1 to 2 tablets per day every 4 hours and keep the patient's daily acetaminophen intake under the 4000 mg maximum daily intake level. Over-the-counter acetaminophen-containing products are not affected by this requirement.

When using acetaminophen for treatment of low back pain, dosing should start at the maximal recommended doses. A typical dosing regimen for acetaminophen would be 1000 mg orally every 6 hours, with a maximum daily dose of 4000 mg.[5,8] Maximum doses should be used for the shortest time possible to minimize occurrence of adverse events.

The adverse effect of greatest concern with acetaminophen is liver toxicity. Data from surveillance programs show that in an 8-year period (1990–1998) there were around 56,000 visits to emergency rooms, 26,000 hospitalizations, and 458 deaths due to acetaminophen overdoses.[13] Consumption of alcohol-containing products while using acetaminophen products increases the risk of liver toxicity. Patients who consume alcohol or have concurrent liver toxicity need to limit their daily acetaminophen intake to 2000 mg.

Nonsteroidal Anti-Inflammatory Drugs

NSAIDs are another option for the treatment of low back pain. Research supports the use of NSAIDs over placebo as treatment for acute back pain.[14] For chronic pain, the data are less convincing. In comparing NSAIDs with acetaminophen, NSAIDs have proved to be more effective but with more risks attached.[14] Clinicians should consider NSAIDs for the treatment of low back pain if a patient fails to respond to acetaminophen after an appropriate trial period.[8]

Clinicians today can choose from a wide variety of different NSAIDs on the market (**Table 1**) to treat low back pain.[15] If a drug from one class does not provide relief, another agent from a different class could be tested for efficacy in the patient. Similar to acetaminophen, maximal recommended doses should be initially prescribed. The use of aspirin cannot be recommended because there are insufficient data to support or refute its use as a treatment for low back pain.[8] No evidence exists that

Table 1
NSAIDs commonly used to treat low back pain

Class/Drug	Oral Dosing
Propionic Acid Derivatives	
Ibuprofen	200–400 mg every 4–6 h (maximum dose 3200 mg)
Naproxen	250 mg 3 to 4 times daily
Acetic Acid Derivatives	
Sulindac	150–200 mg twice daily
Etodolac	200–400 mg 3 to 4 times daily (maximum 1000 mg/d)
Ketorolac	10 mg every 4–6 h (maximum 40 mg/d for no more than 5 d)
Diclofenac	50 mg 3 times daily (maximum 150 mg)
Enolic Acid Derivatives	
Piroxicam	10–20 mg daily to twice daily (maximum 20 mg)
Meloxicam	7.5–15 mg/d (maximum 15 mg)
Nabumetone	500–1000 mg daily to twice daily (maximum 2000 mg)
Cyclooxygenase-2 Selective Inhibitors	
Celecoxib	100–200 mg daily or twice daily

cyclooxygenase-2 inhibitors (Celecoxib, Celebrex) for low back pain treatment provides any additional efficacy compared with traditional NSAIDs.[14]

Safety issues, mainly renal and gastrointestinal toxicities, involving the use of NSAIDs must be considered when deciding to prescribe this class of drugs for low back pain. NSAID-induced acute renal failure ranks second only to aminoglycoside-induced acute renal failure.[16] NSAID-induced acute renal failure accounts for about 15% of all drug-induced renal failure. Nephrotoxicity occurs mainly as a result of prostaglandin inhibition and is usually, but not always, reversible.[16] Interstitial nephritis can occur, which can lead to permanent kidney damage.[16] Gastrointestinal toxicity, also resulting from prostaglandin inhibition, occurs at a rate of 1% to 2% of all NSAID use.[17] Cyclooxygenase-2 inhibitors may have fewer gastrointestinal toxicities in comparison with traditional NSAIDs.[18] If a traditional NSAID is selected for treatment, strategies to prevent NSAID-induced gastrointestinal toxicities include combining NSAID therapy with misoprostol, H2-receptor blockers, or proton-pump inhibitors.[18]

In addition, concern exists for the use of NSAIDs and subsequent cardiovascular toxicity, mainly myocardial infarction. According to the literature, the risk appears to be increased over that of nonusers.[19–22] In general, for patients at increased risk of cardiovascular toxicities, ibuprofen, diclofenac, and meloxicam should be avoided.[19–22] Naproxen is the drug of choice, as it appears that it does not increase the risk of cardiovascular events.[19–22] Because of potential renal, gastrointestinal, and cardiovascular concerns, NSAIDs should be used for the shortest treatment period possible to potentially minimize these concerns.

Tramadol

Only after the patient has failed acetaminophen and NSAID therapy should tramadol be considered an option for the treatment of low back pain.[4,8,23] Tramadol exhibits weak opioid effects and inhibits serotonin and norepinephrine reuptake. Short-term improvements in pain and function have been demonstrated for tramadol (dosed at 50 mg, maximum 400 mg per day for 4 weeks) in the treatment of low back pain, but there is a lack of long-term data.[24] Two studies report that tramadol (37.5 mg) in combination with acetaminophen (325 mg) report improvements in pain in two 3-month trials.[24] Major side effects, occurring at a rate greater than 10%, associated with tramadol include dizziness, nausea, sedation, constipation, and headache.[25] Tramadol use at or above recommended doses has also been associated with seizures.[25] Patients receiving serotonin reuptake inhibitors (SSRIs), tricyclic antidepressants, monoamine oxidase inhibitors, neuroleptics, or other opioids have an even higher potential for occurrence of seizures.[25] Tramadol has a large number of drug interactions, many involving the cytochrome P450 enzyme system (2B6, 2D6, and 3A4).[25] If a clinician is considering prescribing tramadol for a patient with low back pain, it would be prudent to perform a complete review of medication to avoid the possibility of drug interactions. Tramadol use should be avoided in patients with a history of opioid addiction, as reinitiation of physical dependence to opioids can occur.[25] Clinicians should be alert to signs of dependence and abuse among patients using tramadol, even if there is no prior history of opioid dependence.

Opioids

Opioids often are prescribed inappropriately as a first-line therapy for the treatment of low back pain. Opioid use in long-term therapy for chronic low back pain seems to be increasing at an alarming rate, even though the benefits and risks for using these drugs for the treatment of low back pain is lacking.[23] Long-term use of opioids in the treatment of low back pain is not recommended.[8] A Cochrane review of opioids for chronic low back pain only identified one trial, in which opioids were compared with naproxen.[24] Evidence showed that opioids provided greater pain relief and improve mood better than NSAIDs, but patient activity levels were not improved. Opioids exhibit a variety of adverse effects, mainly central nervous system related (drowsiness, dizziness, confusion), cardiovascular (bradycardia, hypotension), and gastrointestinal (constipation and nausea).[26] In addition, they have a high potential for abuse, misuse, and addiction.

Instead of a first-line therapy for low back pain, opioids are more appropriately prescribed as either second-line or third-line therapy for severe, acute back pain.[8] Patients who have significantly reduced quality of life owing to their low back pain, or those with nonsurgical pathology for their back pain, may benefit from opioid treatment.[8]

If opioids are selected as part of the treatment plan for a patient with low back pain, it would be prudent to follow the World Health Organization stepwise pain treatment algorithm, starting with weak opioid/acetaminophen combination product and progressing to a strong opioid if the patient fails an adequate trial of the weak opioid.[27] The selection of which opioid to use should be determined by obtaining a thorough patient history to elicit past opioid use and response to therapy, coexisting health disorders, allergies, concurrent drugs, and financial constraints.

Morphine is considered to be the gold standard for pain management and should be used unless there is a contraindication for its use.[26] Transitioning among different opioids is possible, and current recommendations for equipotent dosing are listed in **Table 2**.[26] If a patient cannot tolerate morphine, a different opioid can be selected. Although there is no ceiling dose for opioids, the guidelines for the use of opioid therapy for chronic pain suggest that if a maximum dose of 120 to 180 mg of morphine (or equivalent) is reached, the patient should be referred to a pain management clinic before further escalating the opioid dose.[9]

When prescribing chronic opioid therapy, the clinician should require the patient to sign a pain contract or opioid agreement that defines the rules patients must follow to take these drugs safely. Common requirements of pain contracts include submitting to random urine and blood drug tests, using only one pharmacy to obtain medications,

Table 2
Commonly used opioid equipotent dosing

Drug	Equianalgesic Oral Dose (mg)	Oral Starting Dose (mg)	Dosing Interval
Morphine	30	30	Every 3–4 h
Hydromorphone	7.5	6	Every 3–4 h
Hydrocodone	30	10	Every 3–4 h
Oxycodone	30	10	Every 3–4 h
Methadone[a]	—	2.5–15	Every 6–12 h

[a] Care should be taken when selecting methadone for treatment of pain, especially when escalating the doses, as there is a tendency for the drug to accumulate with repeated dosing. The patient should be monitored frequently on methadone initiation.

and obtaining prescriptions from only one provider. Contracts often state that if these requirements are not followed, the physician reserves the right to terminate care of the patient. The use of pain contracts is spurred by recent issues with opioid diversion.

Muscle Relaxants

Two categories of muscle relaxants exist. Antispastic agents (baclofen, tizanidine, dantrolene, and diazepam) carry an indication for spasticity related to injury to the central nervous system (ie, multiple sclerosis) and are not recommended for treatment of low back pain.[23] The other category, antispasmodic agents (cyclobenzaprine, methocarbamol, carisoprodol, metaxalone) can be added to treatment plans for low back pain if patients do not respond adequately to first-line analgesics.[23] These agents should be used for the shortest time possible, preferably for no more than 2 weeks in total. Compared with placebo, muscle relaxants show better efficacy in reducing pain and relieving symptoms,[28] but are less effective than NSAIDs, and patients who use muscle relaxants incur the possibility of more side effects from this class of drugs.[28] The major side effects associated with muscle relaxants are related to the central nervous system, mainly sedation and dizziness. The different skeletal muscle relaxants are not pharmacologically related, therefore various drugs may exhibit different efficacy and safety profiles in a patient. The major metabolite of carisoprodol is meprobamate, which exhibits abuse and overdose issues.[29] There is a black-box warning associated with dantrolene use for potentially fatal hepatotoxicity,[30] and tizanidine has reports of reversible hepatotoxicity associated with its use.[31] Selection of which muscle relaxant to use should be based on adverse effects, drug interactions, and cost. Three of the muscle relaxants (carisoprodol, meprobamate, and cyclobenzaprine) are listed on the Beers list of inappropriate medications for older adults (≥65 years).[32] These medications should be avoided in older adults if possible. Of the muscle relaxants available, the most research exists for cyclobenzaprine and tizanidine.[8,23] If the decision is made to use a muscle relaxant for treatment of low back pain, cyclobenzaprine should be considered first, because of the risk of hepatotoxicity with tizanidine use.

Antidepressants

Antidepressants may be prescribed for the treatment of chronic low back pain, but are not an appropriate choice for acute low back pain.[8] The pain relief associated with antidepressants is theorized to be due to the excess norepinephrine in the synapses rather than from the serotonin reuptake inhibition, therefore to treat chronic low back pain it would be sensible to select antidepressants that contain norepinephrine reuptake inhibition as part of the mechanism of action.[8] Randomized clinical trials demonstrate that tricyclic antidepressants (amitriptyline, nortriptyline, desipramine), which exhibit some norepinephrine reuptake inhibition, offer some pain reduction in patients without clinical depression, but no studies have been done in patients who suffer from comorbid depression.[33] Functional improvement did not occur, and greater than 20% of the patients had side effects. In clinical trials, SSRIs failed to be more beneficial than placebo for the treatment of low back pain.[33] Antidepressants with both norepinephrine and serotonin reuptake inhibition, namely duloxetine, venlafaxine, and bupropion, have achieved pain reduction for certain conditions (ie, peripheral neuropathy) but have rarely been studied for treatment of low back pain.[34] Three trials have studied duloxetine for the treatment of chronic low back pain.[35–37] Marginal improvements were seen in 2 of these trials, and in the third no difference was observed. All 3 trials included comparison with placebo, had a significant placebo effect, and were sponsored by the pharmaceutical company that makes the drug.

Antidepressant medications may be helpful in treating patients with low back pain who also suffer from depression.[4,8] Upward of 50% of patients with chronic low back pain exhibit depressive symptoms. It is essential that the treatment plan for low back pain include the treatment of depression, if present, as patients who receive treatment for both conditions have better outcomes.

Benzodiazepines are not recommended to be used for chronic low back pain.[28] These agents portray similar efficacy to skeletal muscle relaxants for acute low back pain, but should not be used for more than 3 or 4 weeks in total. Risks for abuse, addiction, and tolerance outweigh the potential benefit of benzodiazepines for the treatment of low back pain.

Antipsychotic Drugs

Preclinical studies in humans theorize that excessive dopamine may be linked with pain syndromes.[38] It would therefore be reasonable to investigate antipsychotics as an option for pain management. A recent Cochrane review examined the use of antipsychotics for acute and chronic pain in adults.[38] The purpose of the review was to examine efficacy and adverse effects of this drug class in acute or chronic pain. Eleven studies were identified and reviewed, but none of them involved patients with acute or chronic low back pain specifically. Six studies focused on chronic pain management, mainly for cancer pain, headaches, and neuralgic pain. The evidence did not strongly support the use of antipsychotics for chronic pain treatment, even when the trials were combined in a meta-analysis. Many of these trials used first-generation antipsychotics (ie, fluphenazine, thioridazine, prochlorperazine, haloperidol), and none investigated second-generation agents.

Because of the risks and adverse effects associated with antipsychotic drugs, the potential problems with this drug class outweigh the benefits of their use. Adverse effects seen with first-generation antipsychotics include cardiovascular events (QT prolongation, arrhythmias, and so forth), central nervous system events (dystonic reactions, akathisia, extrapyramidal reactions, and so forth), and endocrine events (glucose irregularities and sexual dysfunction). Without confirmed evidence showing efficacy for treatment of low back pain, antipsychotics should not be recommended as therapy. Research involving second-generation antipsychotics may provide evidence for their use, but at present there is none.

Antiseizure Medications

Gabapentin and carbamazepine, both anticonvulsants, have been used to treat chronic low back pain and have been proved to be efficacious for the treatment of sciatica.[4] Gabapentin has a high affinity for voltage-gated calcium channels, which may modulate the release of excitatory neurotransmitters that affect nociception.[39] Carbamazepine has antineuralgic and muscle-relaxant properties and may depress synaptic transmission by limiting sodium-ion influx.[40] Its exact mechanism for pain relief is unknown. Neither agent has been shown to be efficacious for the treatment of chronic low back pain, and therefore cannot be recommended. Pregabalin works in a similar way to gabapentin. Evidence from studies shows that pregabalin, when added to other treatments for low back pain, may provide additional benefit.[41]

Systemic Steroids

Systemic steroids cannot be recommended as a treatment for low back pain, as there is no evidence that demonstrates a benefit from their use.[8] Steroid epidurals are sometimes used as a treatment, and are discussed elsewhere in this issue.

NOVEL THERAPIES

Small clinical trials exist involving the use of a lidocaine 5% patch for the treatment of low back pain. The largest trial (6-week, open-label, nonrandomized) with 77 patients documented that 58% of patients were satisfied or very satisfied with the lidocaine patch for treatment of low back pain.[42] Patients with low back pain of varying severity wore between 1 and 4 patches daily. Assessments completed at 2 and 6 weeks documented improvement in pain intensity and pain interference with quality of life, with minimal to moderate side effects, mainly dizziness and rash. At present, with only minimal published literature available regarding the use of lidocaine 5% patches for the treatment of low back pain, this therapeutic option should be reserved for use when other options have failed to help the patient achieve optimal pain relief. These patches would not be an option in patients with hepatic disease, as these patients are at a higher risk of lidocaine toxicity due to their inability to metabolize the drug normally. Further research using the lidocaine 5% patch is warranted.

ON THE HORIZON

The May Day Fund published proceedings from a 2009 meeting that focused on chronic pain care in the United States (http://www.maydaypainreport.org/docs/A Call to Revolutionize Chronic Pain Care in America 03.04.10.pdf).[3] The convened panel included pain experts from a variety of health disciplines. Their report included 9 action steps to improve the care of patients who suffer from chronic pain. The panel states that current research in the care of pain patients accounts for less than 1% of the budget of the National Institutes of Health (NIH), whereas diabetes research receives about 4% of their funds. Because the number of Americans who suffer from chronic pain tops 116 million (more than cancer, heart disease, and diabetes combined),[43] the panel recommended that the NIH increase the level of funding proportional to the number of people who suffer from chronic pain. Areas starting with basic research and leading to comparative effectiveness studies need to be conducted, with a special emphasis on pain prevention. Because approximately 20% of the nation's children suffer from chronic pain and, as such, they are often undertreated for their pain, research should also focus on ways to prevent childhood pain from becoming a life-long problem.[3]

The Institute of Medicine (IOM) published the report *Relieving Pain in America: A Blueprint for Transforming Prevention, Care, Education, and Research*.[43] In this blueprint, the IOM recommends that the NIH designate a lead institute to move pain research forward and that there should be increased support for multidisciplinary and longitudinal pain research. Furthermore, the report recommends that the Secretary of Health and Human Services create a comprehensive population health-level strategy for pain prevention, treatment, management, and research. The IOM recommends improvement in the process for developing new agents for pain control, including research in new and faster ways for the FDA to evaluate and improve new pain therapies.

Both reports[3,43] recommend that appropriate training and education occur as part of health professions' training programs to adequately equip health care providers with the knowledge needed to appropriately treat patients who suffer from chronic pain. The Mayday Report also states that public education about the risks of untreated and undertreated pain and its prevention be afforded high priority to enhance wellness and diminish the chronic pain crisis in the United States country. By accomplishing these goals, it is hoped that the reliance on opioid therapy by the primary care physician as a treatment for chronic pain will subside.

REFERENCES

1. Prevalence and most common causes of disability among adults—United States, 2005. MMWR Morb Mortal Wkly Rep 2009;58(16):421–6. Available at: http://www.cdc.gov/mmwr/preview/mmwrhtml/mm5816a2.htm. Accessed February 8, 2012.
2. AAPM facts and figures on pain. American Academy of Pain Medicine; 2012. Available at: http://www.painmed.org/patient/facts.html. Accessed February 8, 2012.
3. A call to revolutionize chronic pain care in America: an opportunity in health care reform. The Mayday Fund; 2012. Available at: http://www.maydaypainreport.org/docs/A%20Call%20to%20Revolutionize%20Chronic%20Pain%20Care%20in%20America%2003.04.10.pdf. Accessed February 8, 2012.
4. Duffy RL. Low back pain: an approach to diagnosis and management. Prim Care Clin Office Pract 2010;37:729–41.
5. Kincade S. Evaluation and treatment of acute low back pain. Am Fam Physician 2007;75:1181–8.
6. Laine C, Goldmann D, Wilson JF. In the clinic: low back pain. Arch Intern Med 2008;148. ITC5-1–ITC5-16.
7. Last AR, Kulber K. Chronic low back pain: evaluation and management. Am Fam Physician 2009;79:1067–74.
8. Chou R, Qaseem A, Snow V, et al. Diagnosis and treatment of low back pain: a joint clinical practice guideline from the American College of Physicians and the American Pain Society. Ann Intern Med 2007;147:478–91.
9. Chou R, Fanciullo GJ, Fine PG, et al. Clinical guidelines for the use of chronic opioid therapy for chronic noncancer pain. J Pain 2009;10:113–30.
10. Deyo RA, Weinstein JN. Low back pain. N Engl J Med 2001;344:363–70.
11. Williams CM, Latimer J, Maher CG, et al. PACE—the first placebo controlled trial of paracetamol for acute low back pain: design of a randomized controlled trial. BMC Musculoskelet Disord 2010;11:169.
12. Questions and answers about oral prescription acetaminophen products to be limited to 321 mg per dosage unit. Food and Drug Administration; 2012. Available at: http://www.fda.gov/Drugs/DrugSafety/InformationbyDrugClass/ucm239871.htm. Accessed February 8, 2012.
13. Nourjah P, Ahmad SR, Karwoski C, et al. Estimates of acetaminophen (paracetamol)-associated overdoses in the United States. Pharmacoepidemiol Drug Saf 2006;15:398–405.

14. Roelofs PD, Deyo RA, Koes BW, et al. Non-steroidal anti-inflammatory drugs for low back pain. Cochrane Database Syst Rev 2008;(1):CD000396.
15. Burke A, Smyth E, FitzGerald GA. Analgesic-antipyretic agents; pharmacotherapy of gout. In: Brunton L, Lazo J, Parker K, editors. Goodman & Gilman's the pharmacological basis of therapeutics. 11th edition. New York: McGraw – Hill; 2006. p. 671–717.
16. Ejaz P, Bhojani K, Joshi VR. NSAIDs and kidney. J Assoc Physicians India 2004; 52:632–40.
17. Cryer B. NSAID-associated deaths: the rise and fall of NSAID-associated GI mortality. Am J Gastroenterol 2005;100:1694–5.
18. Rostom A, Muir K, Dube C, et al. Prevention of NSAID-related upper gastrointestinal toxicity: a meta-analysis of traditional NSAIDs with gastroprotection and COX-2 inhibitors. Drug Healthc Patient Saf 2009;1:47–71.
19. Fosbol EL, Folke F, Jacobson S, et al. Cause-specific cardiovascular risk associated with nonsteroidal antiinflammatory drugs among healthy individuals. Circ Cardiovasc Qual Outcomes 2010;3:395–405.
20. Graham DJ. COX-2 inhibitors, other NSAIDs, and cardiovascular risk: the seduction of common sense. JAMA 2006;296:1653–6.
21. Ray WA, Varas-Lorenzo C, Chung CP, et al. Cardiovascular risks of nonsteroidal anti-inflammatory drugs in patients after hospitalization for serious coronary heart disease. Circ Cardiovasc Qual Outcomes 2009;2:155–63.
22. McGettigan P, Henry D. Cardiovascular risk and inhibition of cyclooxygenase: a systematic review of the observational studies of select and nonselective inhibitors of cyclooxygenase-2. JAMA 2006;296:1633–44.
23. Lee T. Pharmacologic treatment for low back pain: one component of pain care. Phys Med Rehabil Clin N Am 2010;21:793–800.
24. Deshpande A, Furlan AD, Mailis-Gagnon A, et al. Opioids for chronic low-back pain. Cochrane Database Syst Rev 2007;(3):CD004959.
25. Lexicomp online. Tramadol. Hudson (OH): Lexi-Comp Inc; 2012.
26. Gutstein HB, Akil H. Opioid analgesics. In: Brunton L, Lazo J, Parker K, editors. Goodman & Gilman's the pharmacological basis of therapeutics. 11th edition. New York: McGraw – Hill; 2006. p. 547–91.
27. WHO's pain ladder. HO stepwise pain management. World Health Organization; 2012. Available at: http://www.who.int/cancer/palliative/painladder/en/. Accessed February 8, 2012.
28. van Tulder MW, Touray T, Furlan AD, et al. Muscle relaxants for non-specific low-back pain. Cochrane Database Syst Rev 2003;(4):CD004252.
29. Lexicomp online. Carisoprodal. Hudson (OH): Lexi-Comp Inc; 2012.
30. Lexicomp online. Dantrolene. Hudson (OH): Lexi-Comp Inc; 2012.
31. Lexicomp online. Tizanidine. Hudson (OH): Lexi-Comp Inc; 2012.
32. Fick DM, Cooper JW, Wade WE, et al. Updating the Beers criteria for potentially inappropriate medication use in older adults: results of a US consensus panel of experts. Arch Intern Med 2003;163:2716–24.
33. Urquhart DM, Hoving JL, Assendelft WJ, et al. Antidepressants for non-specific low back pain. Cochrane Database Syst Rev 2008;(1):CD001703.
34. Lunn MP, Hughes RA, Wiffen PJ. Duloxetine for treating painful neuropathy or chronic pain. Cochrane Database Syst Rev 2009;(4):CD007115.
35. Skljarevski V, Desaiah D, Liu-Seifert H, et al. Efficacy and safety of duloxetine in patients with chronic low back pain (*CLBP-1*). Spine 2010;35:E578–85.
36. Skljarevski V, Ossanna M, Liu-Seifert H, et al. A double-blind, randomized trial of duloxetine versus placebo in the management of chronic low back pain (*CLBP-2*). Eur J Neurol 2009;16:1041–8.

37. Skljarevski V, Zhang S, Desaiah D, et al. Duloxetine versus placebo in patients with chronic low back pain: a 12-week, fixed-dose, randomized, double-blind trial (*CLBP-3*). J Pain 2010;11:1282–90.

38. Seidel S, Aigner M, Ossege M, et al. Antipsychotics for acute and chronic pain in adults. Cochrane Database Syst Rev 2008;(4).

39. Lexicomp online. Gabapentin. Hudson (OH): Lexi-Comp Inc; 2012.

40. Lexicomp online. Carbamazepine. Hudson (OH): Lexi-Comp Inc; 2012.

41. Romano CL, Romano D, Bonora C, et al. Pregabalin, celecoxib, and their combination for treatment of chronic low back pain. J Orthop Traumatol 2009;10: 185–91.

42. Gimble J, Linn R, Hale M, et al. Lidocaine patch treatment in patients with low back pain: results of an open label, non randomized pilot study. Am J Ther 2005;12:311–9.

43. IOM (Institute of Medicine). Relieving pain in America: a blueprint for transforming prevention, care, education and research. Washington, DC: The National Academies Press; 2011.

Mechanical Therapy for Low Back Pain

Donald Grant Guild, MD

KEYWORDS

- Low back pain • McKenzie method • Mechanical therapy • Ultrasonography

KEY POINTS

- There are a vast variety of techniques that physical therapists commonly use in the treatment of low back pain. Some of the therapies include, but are certainly not limited to education, exercise, lumbar traction, manual manipulation, application of heat, cryotherapy, and ultrasonography.
- The most popular method of physical therapy in the United States and other countries is the McKenzie approach. The principal assumption for the McKenzie method is that patients have pain that centralizes or is extinguished with a lumbar exercise in a single direction.
- Another intervention that is commonly offered to patients in the treatment of low back pain is the thrust manipulation.

The most popular method of physical therapy in the United States and other countries is the McKenzie approach. This approach, developed by Robert McKenzie from New Zealand, bears his name and is known as the McKenzie Method of Mechanical Diagnosis and Therapy (MDT). The method starts by obtaining a detailed history and physical examination by the physical therapist. The physical examination and the history are focused on identifying characteristic patterns of pain in patients, which will guide the physical therapist to an accurate pathoanatomic source of the underlying pain. The principal assumption of the McKenzie method is that patients have pain that centralizes or is extinguished with lumbar exercise in a single direction. Many patients experience prompt pain relief with extension maneuvers and exercise, eliminating the need for analgesic or nonsteroidal anti-inflammatory drugs with certain maneuvers. In this regard, the McKenzie technique differs from other specific lumbar extension exercises because it is does not necessarily always depend on lumbar extension to relieve pain. In theory, the McKenzie method assigns patients to homogeneous groups with similar low back pain. Therefore, the patients are classified according to the centralization phenomenon (directional preference). Specific exercises can then be prescribed to reverse the damage.[1]

Southern Regional AHEC, 1601 Owen Drive, Fayetteville, NC 28304, USA
E-mail address: Donald.guild@sr-ahec.org

Prim Care Clin Office Pract 39 (2012) 511–516
http://dx.doi.org/10.1016/j.pop.2012.06.006
0095-4543/12/$ – see front matter © 2012 Published by Elsevier Inc.

primarycare.theclinics.com

A meta-analysis of randomized controlled trials found that the McKenzie method is effective for low back pain (Strength of Recommendation Taxonomy [SORT] Level B). Eleven trials of mostly high quality were included in the analysis. The McKenzie technique reduced pain (weighted mean difference) on a 0- to 100-point scale by −4.16 points (95% confidence interval [CI] −7.12 to −1.20) and disability by −5.22 (95% CI −8.28 to −2.16) at 1-week follow-up, in a comparison with passive therapy (ie, educational booklets, bed rest, ice packs, and massage).[2]

Another intervention commonly offered to patients in the treatment of low back pain is the thrust manipulation (**Fig. 1**), which involves a standard technique. The patient is placed in the supine position. Next, the patient is passively moved into side-bending mode by the therapist. The therapist is positioned to the opposite side of the patient. The patient is instructed to interlock the fingers behind the head. Finally the therapist thrusts the anterior inferior iliac spine. The direction of the thrust is in the posterior and inferior direction. Both the patient and the therapist listen for a cavitation or "joint pop."[3] Cavitation is theorized to occur when the synovial fluid in the joint space changes from a liquid to a gaseous state. The exact effect of the fluid is unknown.[4] The manipulation is attempted again if no cavitation is heard or experienced by the patient. If a cavitation is not heard on the second attempt, the maneuver is repeated on the opposite side. If a cavitation is heard, the patient is instructed on range-of-motion exercises.[3] The thrust is very similar to the procedure used by chiropractors and osteopathic physicians using manipulation therapy.

APPLICATION OF HEAT AND COLD

Application of heat produces a variety of physiologic effects. Heat cause vasodilation of vessels resulting in a 2- to 3-fold increase in blood flow to the region, which allows for increased nutrients, antibodies, and leukocytes, and increased removal of metabolic byproducts. This process may contribute to edema in the region. Therefore, heat is usually best used for chronic inflammatory conditions rather than for acute low back pain. Heat has been shown to maximize tendon extensibility and to promote

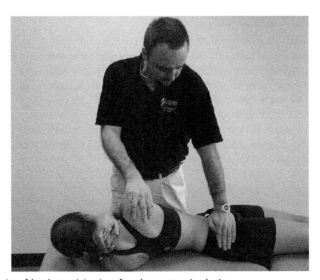

Fig. 1. Example of body positioning for thrust manipulation.

healing. Heat has a generally relaxing effect, although its mechanism of action is unknown.

Application of cold causes immediate cutaneous vasoconstriction, which has the effect of decreasing edema in tissues. Cryotherapy reduces the velocity of nerve conduction, thus decreasing the sensation of pain. Prolonged cold exposure causes cessation of axonal-plasmic transport and axonal degeneration. Cold may slow the process of collagenolysis in inflammatory arthropathies.[5]

Based on a meta-analysis that reviewed a total of 1117 different patients for the effectiveness of application of hot and cold to low back pain, there is limited evidence to recommend either (SORT B). Heat treatments included hot-water bottles, soft heated backs with grains, hot towels, heating pads, infrared heat lamps, saunas, steam, electric heating blankets, heat wraps, ultrasound, heated stones, and hot baths. There is moderate evidence that a heat wrap reduces pain and disability for patients with back pain that lasts for less than 3 months. The effect seemed to be limited to a short time and the effect was relatively small. In this meta-analysis, treatment of acute injury included cold towels, cold gel packs, ice packs, and ice massage. There was even more limited evidence for the effectiveness of cold in the treatment of low back pain.[6]

PHYSICAL CONDITIONING AND EXERCISES

Exercise therapy is widely used as a treatment modality for nonspecific low back pain. A meta-analysis that examined at 61 randomized controlled trials with a total of 6390 patients reported slight evidence that exercise therapy reduced pain, decreased absenteeism, and improved function (SORT B).[7]

There have been 8 studies comparing patients with low back pain on exercise protocol with others on the waiting list or under no treatment. There was no statistical difference in the overall reduction in pain and improvement of disability (SORT Level C).[8]

A total of 6 studies were done on the treatment of low back pain with exercise therapy versus the "usual care and advice to stay active." Three of the studies demonstrated a statistically significant reduction in reported pain and disability. There was a statistical difference for disability in the groups that received exercise therapy. The magnitude of the effect was a reduction of 9.23 (95% CI −16.02 to −2.643) and 12.35 (95% CI −23.00 to −1.69), respectively, on scale of 1 to 100 (SORT B).[9] One study compared the percentage of patients that reported recovery at 3 months. The group that was prescribed exercise therapy compared with the usual care group was found to have higher percentage of recovery 80% versus 47% respectively (SORT C).[10]

In a comparison of exercise versus back school/education, four studies were pooled. The data were noted to be of poor quality owing to study design and data-collection flaws. There was no statistically significant effect on pain or disability of the exercise groups in comparison with back school/education (SORT C).[9]

In summary, no significant differences were seen with exercise treatment groups in comparison with waiting-list and no-treatment groups. However, exercise therapy did show a significant improvement in both pain and disability when compared with usual care at short-term follow-up.

TRANSCUTANEOUS ELECTRICAL NERVE STIMULATION

The transcutaneous electrical nerve stimulation (TENS) unit applies an electrical current to the nerve endings by application of electrodes to the skin. TENS stimulates proprioceptive nerve fibers, which generate special-location data or A fibers. This topic is reviewed in an article elsewhere in this issue. The vast number of A fibers stimulated is thought to block the transition of pain signals or C fibers by overloading dorsal ganglion laminae, which act as a gatekeeper in the spinal cord. The T fibers that originate in the substantia gelatinosa then effectively block the pain signal from reaching the thalamus were pain is perceived. Researchers have found that they can selectively stimulate A fibers without stimulating C fibers by using phasic input. The C fibers tend to react more to continuous waveforms or those perceived as continuous by the brain. There is another theory that TENS units work by increasing the release of endogenous endorphin molecules.[11]

A total of 5 studies compared the effectiveness of TENS with sham treatment. A meta-analysis of pooled data from 2 studies found no statistically significant difference in disability. One study with a low risk of bias did demonstrate a greater effect on pain intensity with the TENS treatment groups than with the sham-TENS group.[9] It is therefore difficult to determine an evidence-based recommendation for the use of TENS units for the treatment of low back pain. The risk-benefit ratio is in favor of patient treatment with low associated side effects and cost, therefore it is a reasonable option. However, further well-designed studies are necessary before a recommendation can be made.

MASSAGE

Massage is thought to stimulate the nervous system and the endocrine system. Massage moves body fluids and has a direct effect on connective tissues. It is thought that massage causes the brain to increase the concentration of endorphin and norendorphin, which are pain-relieving hormones. Moreover, in response to massage the body produces several opiate-like compounds. Enkephalin and β-endorphins bind opioid receptors, helping to alleviate chronic pain and acute pain, and producing euphoria.

Dopamine has also been found to increase in response to massage. Dopamine is involved in a variety of emotions and behaviors and is well known to influence motor activity, the ability to focus, learn, and moods such as inspiration, joy, and enthusiasm. Lack of dopamine has been known to cause contrary effects (lack of motor control, poor attention, and boredom).[12] An exact correlation between dopamine and pain relief with massage, however, has not been demonstrated.

A meta-analysis of 13 randomized trials with a total of 1596 patients was done to determine the effectiveness of massage therapy for low back pain. Massage worked more often when paired with exercise therapy or stretching. The benefits were greater when compared with mobilization, relaxation, physical therapy, self care, and education. No serious adverse events were reported. Some patients did experience some soreness after therapy. Massage may be beneficial to patients with low back pain lasting as long as 4 to 12 weeks or pain lasting longer than 12 weeks (SORT A).[13]

Three studies compared massage therapy with acupuncture and relaxation therapy. However, there was a high risk of bias in the study design. There was no statistically significant reduction in pain intensity in the massage group compared with the control groups (SORT C).[9]

TRACTION

Axial traction has been used for centuries as a treatment for low back pain. It was first popularized by Crisp and colleagues[14] as an intervention for patients with nerve root involvement due to lumbar intervertebral disk herniation (SORT C).

The most common types of traction used to treat subacute and chronic low back pain with and without sciatica are mechanical or motorized traction. In the latter system the traction is exerted by a motorized pulley with the patient secured to a traction table. Alternatively, the therapist uses his or her body weight to generate the forces and direction of the traction.

A meta-analysis was completed to determine the effectiveness of traction for low back pain. Included were 25 trials with a total of 2206 patients with low back pain. Traction was consistently no more effective than placebo, regardless of whether it was continuous or intermittent. There were reports of adverse effects in some patients who received intermittent or continuous traction. Some patients experienced increased pain and subsequent surgery (SORT C).[15]

LUMBAR SUPPORTS

In a review of randomized controlled trials a total of 13,995 patients with lumbar supports, also known as corsets, were assessed for the effect on prevention of low back pain and treatment. Little to no evidence was found that lumbar support prevented back injury more than education on proper lifting technique. The review included 954 patients in a comparison of lumbar supports with no treatment for prevention of low back pain, with similar results. There was little to no evidence to support their use for prevention of low back injury. An individual study did show that lumbar supports did decrease the number of sick days but not prevention of back pain. In summary, there was some weak evidence that lumbar supports help in the treatment of low back pain, given that patients had a decreased number of sick days.

In a review of 14 studies including 1170 patients who had acute and chronic low back pain, there was minimal to no difference in pain between the use of lumbar supports and no treatment. A review of the data from 2 studies including 550 patients reported that there was conflicting evidence as to whether lumbar supports helped patients regain functional status and return to work sooner.

In 3 studies that included a total of 954 patients, there was no significant difference in pain or decrease in the number of days before return to work with the use of lumbar supports when compared with patients who received physiotherapy, manipulation, or electrical stimulation (SORT C).[16]

REFERENCES

1. Kinkade S. Evaluation and treatment of acute low back pain [Letters to the Editor]. Am Fam Physician 2008;77–748.
2. Carneiro LA, de Souza MS. The McKenzie method for low back pain. A systemic review of the literature with a meta-analysis approach. Spine 2006;31:E254–62.
3. Cleland JA, Fritz JM. Comparison of the effectiveness of three manual physical therapy techniques in a subgroup of patients with low back pain who satisfy a clinical prediction rule: study protocol of a randomized clinical trial. BMC Musculoskelet Disord 2006;7(11):1471–2474.
4. DeStefano L. Greenman's principles of manual medicine. 4th edition; 2011.
5. DeStenafo L. Principles of manual medicine. 4th edition; 2011.
6. Superficial heat or cold for low back pain (review). The Cochrane Collaboration; 2011.
7. Hayden J, van Tulder MW. Exercise therapy for treatment of non-specific low back pain (review). 2011.
8. Smeets RJ, Vlaeyen JW, Hidding A, et al. Active rehabilitation for chronic low back pain: cognitive-behavioral, physical, or both? First direct post-treatment results from a randomized controlled trial. BMC Musculoskelet Disord 2006;7:5.

9. Middelkoop M, Rubinstein SM. A systemic review of the effectiveness of physical and rehabilitation interventions for chronic non-specific low back pain. Eur Spine J 2011;20(1):19–23.

10. Niemisto L, Murphy B. Self-report measures best explain changes in disability compared with physical measures after exercise rehabilitation for chronic low back pain. Spine 2008;33:326–38.

11. Kahn J. Principles and practice of electrotherapy. 4th edition; 2000. p. 101–3.

12. Fritz JM, Thackeray A, Childs JD, et al. A randomized clinical trial of the effectiveness of mechanical traction for sub-groups of patients with low back pain: methods and rationale. BMC Musculoskelet Disord 2011;11:81.

13. Massage for low-back pain (review). The Cochrane Collaboration; 2011.

14. Crisp EJ, Cyriax JH, Cristie BG. Discussion on the treatment of backache by traction. Proc R Soc Med 1955;48:805–14.

15. Traction for low-back pain with or without sciatica (review). The Cochrane Collaboration; 2011.

16. Lumbar supports for the prevention and treatment of low back pain (review). The Cochrane Collaboration; 2011.

Nonsurgical Interventions for Low Back Pain

Harkiran Grewal, MD[a],*, Bikramjit S. Grewal, MD[b], Rashita Patel, MD[a]

KEYWORDS

- Low back pain • Interventions • Nonsurgical • Therapy

KEY POINTS

- Despite low back pain being a self-limiting condition, there are a variety of therapeutic interventions, including nonsurgical modalities available for management of chronic low back pain, such as injections, irritants, proteolytic enzymes, laser therapy, radiofrequency denervation, intradiscal electrothermal therapy, percutaneous intradiscal radiofrequency thermoregulation, and coblation nucleoplasty.
- According to the American Pain Society, Medicare-reported rates for spinal epidural injection increased by 271% and facet joint injection by 231% between 1994 and 2001. Given the increase in the application of these procedures, there is no associated improvement in the health status of patients with chronic low back pain. Most of the procedures are based on success stories of individual case studies and observational studies.[1,2]

INTRODUCTION

Despite low back pain being a self-limiting condition, there are a variety of therapeutic interventions available. This article reviews the nonsurgical modalities available for management of chronic low back pain, such as injections, irritants, proteolytic enzymes, laser therapy, radiofrequency denervation, intradiscal electrothermal therapy, percutaneous intradiscal radiofrequency thermoregulation, and coblation nucleoplasty. According to the American Pain Society, Medicare-reported rates for spinal epidural injection increased by 271% and facet joint injection by 231% between 1994 and 2001. Given the increase in the application of these procedures, there is no associated improvement in the health status of patients with chronic low back pain. Most of the procedures are based on success stories of individual case studies and observational studies.[1,2]

INJECTIONS
Injection Therapy

Injection therapy has long been in use for subacute and chronic low back pain. Injections are given into different locations, such as spinal facet joints, epidural space,

[a] Southern Regional AHEC, 1601 Owen Drive, Fayetteville, NC 28304, USA; [b] University of Chapel Hill, NC, USA
* Corresponding author.
E-mail address: harkiran.grewal@sr-ahec.org

Prim Care Clin Office Pract 39 (2012) 517–523
http://dx.doi.org/10.1016/j.pop.2012.06.007
0095-4543/12/$ – see front matter © 2012 Published by Elsevier Inc.

primarycare.theclinics.com

spinal nerve roots, local ligaments, and sacroiliac joints, using different pharmacologic agents such as corticosteroids, anesthetic agents, nonsteroidal antiinflammatory drugs (NSAIDs), and opioids, alone or in combination.[3] Injections are classified into nonspinal versus spinal injections depending on where the substance is injected. There are range of adverse effects of injections including headaches, dizziness, transient local pain, nausea, and vomiting to more severe effects such as septic facet joint arthritis,[4] paraspinal abscess,[5] discitis,[6] and cauda equina syndrome.[7]

Nonspinal Injections

Nonspinal injections include:

Botulinum toxin injection

Botulinum toxin (BoNT) is an antispasmodic that is injected into the muscles of the back. BoNT is produced by *Clostridium botulinum*, a gram-positive anaerobic bacterium. BoNT acts by binding presynaptically to high-affinity recognition sites on the cholinergic nerve terminals and suppressing the release of acetylcholine, causing a neuromuscular blocking effect. This mechanism laid the foundation for the development of the toxin as a therapeutic tool. BoNT injection is increasingly being used as a therapeutic modality for the treatment of low back pain. Some of the commercial names of BoNT include Botox, Lantox, Myobloc, and Neurobloc. The Cochrane Review[8] was of BoNT injections for patients with nonspecific low back pain (ie, back pain without an obvious underlying cause), with or without sciatica. There is little or no evidence that it benefits patients with chronic back pain. The current body of evidence does not support the use of BoNT injections to improve pain or function in patients with low back pain. There is only low-quality evidence that BoNT injections are more effective than saline or corticosteroid injections or acupuncture for reducing low back pain. The present literature has yet to address the long-term benefits of BoNT injections or the cost benefits of this therapy.

Trigger point injections

This is a type of local injection in which substances such as corticosteroid or anesthetics are injected at the point of maximal tenderness, often with a palpable nodule or band. In patients with iliac crest pain syndrome, there is moderate evidence suggesting the effectiveness for short-term pain relief with local anesthetic at the point of maximal tenderness over the medial part of the iliac crest compared with placebo. As for the corticosteroids, patients have reported improvement without any pain relief in the short term with injections in the iliolumbar ligament compared with placebo.[9,10] Intramuscular vitamin B_{12} injections have significant effect on short-term pain relief and disability improvement.[11]

Prolotherapy

Prolotherapy is a procedure in which an irritant chemical is injected into the soft tissues of the back to provoke an inflammatory response that subsequently leads to strengthening of the soft tissues with a decrease in pain and disability. It is also referred to as sclerotherapy. Two randomized controlled trials (RCTs) with 160 patients found that prolotherapy injections were more effective for both chronic pain and disability. Prolotherapy is more effective when used in combination with spinal manipulation, exercise, and other interventions than when used alone.[12]

Spinal Injections

Spinal injections include injection of various substances into the space between the dura and the spinal cord. Corticosteroids, NSAIDs, benzodiazepines, and anesthetics are commonly used. Spinal injections can be further divided into:

Epidural steroid injection

This refers to the injection of corticosteroids via a catheter into the space between the dura and the spinal cord. Common approaches for administering epidural steroid injections are through the interlaminar space, via the neuroforamen under fluoroscopic guidance (transforaminal), and through the sacral hiatus at the sacral canal (caudal). Some small trials comparing corticosteroids with placebo failed to show significant short-term pain relief in the corticosteroid groups.[13] In patients after laminectomy, studies were done using different combinations of corticosteroids versus NSAIDs and/or benzodiazepines, with no significant difference in pain relief or general improvement at 1-month and 6-month intervals.[14–17]

Local anesthetic epidural injections

These have been tried with varying success. Studies of anesthetic agents such as ropivacaine and bupivacaine failed to show a significant difference in the pain scores.[18,19]

Chemonucleolysis

Chemonucleolysis entails the injection of the intradiscal space with proteolytic enzymes. One of the most commonly used enzymes is chymopapain, which is extracted from papaya. Chymopapain digests the jellylike inner portion of the disc known as the nucleus pulposus, leaving the outer portion, the annulus fibrosis, intact.

Facet joint steroid injection

Facet joints, small joints that help to stabilize vertebrae, have also been used as a site for injecting. When comparing corticosteroids versus placebo injection at the facet joint, there was no significant difference in pain, disability, and work attendance at 6-week and 3-month intervals.[20,21] Local anesthetic injections at facet joints in combination with Sarapin (suspension of powdered *Sarracenia purpurea*) failed to show a difference in pain relief; overall health; physical, functional, and psychological status; and return to work at short-term and long-term follow-up, when used alone versus in combination with corticosteroids.[22–25]

Medial nerve block

Medial nerve is a branch of posterior ramus that innervates the facet joints in the spine. Medial nerve blocks are used primarily as a diagnostic procedure to diagnose facet joint disease, but they can also be therapeutic. Other sites of injection include the intradiscal and sacroiliac joints.

LASER THERAPY

Low-level laser therapy has been used by physiotherapists and other health care practitioners in musculoskeletal medicine, which generates light of a single wavelength without emitting heat, sound, or vibration. It does so by photochemical reactions in cells, also known as photobiology.[26,27] The mechanism by which low-level laser therapy is postulated to work is by enhancing the fibroblast function, accelerating connective tissue growth, and through antiinflammatory effects by reduction of prostaglandin synthesis.[28,29] Lasers used in low-level laser are is generally less than 5 mW, class 3a with an output of less than 500 mW.[26] There are several RCTs comparing different laser wavelength treatments with sham laser, indicating that laser therapy is effective at reducing back pain for 3 to 6 months compared with controls. There are insufficient data to support or oppose the use of low-level laser therapy for chronic use in patients with chronic low back pain.

RADIOFREQUENCY DENERVATION

Radiofrequency denervation is a procedure involving the destruction of nerves using heat generated by a radiofrequency current.

INTRADISCAL ELECTROTHERMAL THERAPY

Intradiscal electrothermal therapy (IDET) is the placement within the inner posterior annulus of the disc space of a catheter tipped with a temperature-controlled, thermal-resistive heating coil. The temperature is then increased to a maximum of 90°C and held constant for a few minutes, leading to thermocoagulation of nociceptors and unmyelinated nerve fibers, which ultimately causes collagen shrinking and stabilization of annular fissures. A cohort study by Saal and Saal,[30] following 62 patients, asked patients who received IDET to fill out a Short Form 36 questionnaire. The results showed a mean visual analog score (VAS) decrease from 6.57 to 3.41, average sitting time improved by 52.7 minutes, 81% of the patients showed a 7-point improvement in their daily physical function, and 78% showed a 7-point improvement in pain. In another retrospective study, by Derby and colleagues,[31] 32 patients with IDET treatment of annular fissures and global disc degeneration were reviewed. This study showed that 62.5% of patients with the treatment had favorable outcomes; however, 25% had no change, and 12.5% had an unfavorable outcome. One patient in that study suffered from a persistent back pain and was forced to undergo spinal fusion. However, 2 RCTs[32,33] showed inconsistent evidence on the effectiveness of IDET. A study by Pauza and colleagues[32] showed a positive effect on pain severity only, whereas a study by Freeman and colleagues[33] showed a more substantial benefit from the procedure.

PERCUTANEOUS INTRADISCAL RADIOFREQUENCY THERMOCOAGULATION

Percutaneous intradiscal radiofrequency thermocoagulation (PIRFT) is a procedure involving the placement of an electrode/catheter into the intervertebral disc and applying alternating radiofrequency current. It is sometimes classified as a variant of intradiscal electrothermal therapy. In a nonrandomized comparison of IDET with PIRFT by Kapural and colleagues,[34] on 21 patients per group over 12 months, the mean VAS for patients having IDET decreased from 7.9 before the procedure to 1.4 after the procedure. However, in the patients having PIRFT, the VAS decreased from 6.6 before the procedure to 4.4 after the procedure. These results led to the conclusion that IDET offered better treatment compared with PIRFT, and that PIRFT was not an effective treatment of discogenic low back pain.[35,36]

COBLATION NUCLEOPLASTY

Coblation nucleoplasty is a procedure involving the use of a bipolar radiofrequency current to create a series of channels in an intervertebral disc and reduce the volume of tissue. Nucleoplasty has the advantages of faster recovery, earlier return to work, less operative time, less surgery-related trauma, less significant pain, and fewer complications. Sharps and Isaac[37] did a retrospective study on 42 patients with protuberant lumbar intervertebral discs who received coblation nucleoplasty. Patients had marked improvement in rate of VAS immediately after the procedure, but the improvement waned by the 1-year and 2-year follow-ups. The study participants had 66.2% reduction in back pain, 68.1% reduction in leg pain, and 85.7% reduction in numbness within 1 week of the operation. Within a year, follow-up of the coblation nucleoplasty, they had 53.2% reduction in back pain, 58.4% reduction in leg pain, and 81.0% reduction in numbness. At the 2-year follow-up, those numbers change to 45.5% reduction in back pain, 50.7% reduction in leg pain, and 75.0% reduction in numbness. Although the scores decreased, they were still an improvement from before the treatment, and thus coblation nucleoplasty was considered an efficacious mode of treatment of contained disc herniation. Multiple studies performed on patients who have undergone nucleoplasty have shown marked improvement in symptoms. A study by Masala and colleagues[38] showed a 79% improvement in numeric pain after nucleoplasty. The study by Singh and colleagues[39] of 67 patients showed a 50% reduction of pain scores in 53% of the patient population who underwent nucleoplasty, and the study by Reddy and colleagues[40] of 67 patients showed that 54% of patients in the study reported improvement in pain after 1 year. According to the study by Bhagia and colleagues,[41] the most common side effect reported by patients who underwent nucleoplasty was soreness at the needle insertion site, followed by new onset of neuropathies and pain in the leg, which usually resolved within 2 weeks of the procedure and had no impact on functionality. In contrast, a Cochrane review by Gibson and colleageus[42] on surgical interventions for lumbar disc protrusions found no published RCTs that assessed coblation nucleoplasty. The study states that about 100,000 nucleoplasty procedures have been done worldwide since 2005. Any studies including these patients have been ill-defined cohort studies measuring subjective data with inadequate follow-up. The review considers coblation nucleoplasty to be a research technique because no proper RCTs have been published on the subject. A quasi-RCT performed by Nardi and colleagues[43] performed nucleoplasty on 50 patients with contained disc protrusion in the cervical spine who presented with arm pain and neck pain. Twenty patients were placed in a control group and randomized to receive conservative therapy with antiinflammatory medications, cervical collars, and physical therapy.

SUMMARY

A variety of nonoperative interventions are available for treatment of back pain. Careful assessment, discussion, and planning need to be performed to individualize care to each patient. This article discusses good to fair evidence from RCTs that injection therapy, PIRFT, IDET, and prolotherapy are not effective. Evidence is poor from RCTs regarding local injections, Botox, and coblation nucleoplasty; however, with a focused approach, the right treatment can be provided for the right patient. To be more effective in management of back pain, further high-grade RCTs on efficacy and safety are needed.

REFERENCES

1. Friedly J, Chan L, Deyo R. Increases in lumbosacral injections in the Medicare population: 1994 to 2001. Spine (Phila Pa 1976) 2007;32(16):1754–60.
2. Martin BI, Deyo RA, Mirza SK, et al. Expenditures and health status among adults with back and neck problems. JAMA 2008;299(6):656–64.
3. Airaksinen O, Brox JI, Cedraschi C, et al. Chapter 4. European guidelines for the management of chronic nonspecific low back pain. Eur Spine J 2006;15(Suppl 2): S192–300.
4. Weingarten TN, Hooten WM, Huntoon MA. Septic facet joint arthritis after a corticosteroid facet injection. Pain Med 2006;7(1):52–6.
5. Cook NJ, Hanrahan P, Song S. Paraspinal abscess following facet joint injection. Clin Rheumatol 1999;18(1):52–3.
6. Hooten WM, Mizerak A, Carns PE, et al. Discitis after lumbar epidural corticosteroid injection: a case report and analysis of the case report literature. Pain Med 2006;7(1):46–51.
7. Bilir A, Gulec S. Cauda equina syndrome after epidural steroid injection: a case report. J Manipulative Physiol Ther 2006;29(6):492.e1–3.
8. Waseem Z, Boulias C, Gordon A, et al. Botulinum toxin injections for low-back pain and sciatica. Cochrane Database Syst Rev 2011;1:CD008257.

9. Sonne M, Christensen K, Hansen SE, et al. Injection of steroids and local anaesthetics as therapy for low-back pain. Scand J Rheumatol 1985;14(4):343–5.

10. Garvey TA, Marks MR, Wiesel SW. A prospective, randomized, double-blind evaluation of trigger-point injection therapy for low-back pain. Spine (Phila Pa 1976) 1989;14(9):962–4.

11. Mauro GL, Martorana U, Cataldo P, et al. Vitamin B12 in low back pain: a randomised, double-blind, placebo-controlled study. Eur Rev Med Pharmacol Sci 2000;4(3):53–8.

12. Dagenais S, Yelland MJ, Del Mar C, et al. Prolotherapy injections for chronic low-back pain. Cochrane Database Syst Rev 2007;2:CD004059.

13. Beliveau P. A comparison between epidural anaesthesia with and without corticosteroid in the treatment of sciatica. Rheumatol Phys Med 1971;11(1):40–3.

14. Serrao JM, Marks RL, Morley SJ, et al. Intrathecal midazolam for the treatment of chronic mechanical low back pain: a controlled comparison with epidural steroid in a pilot study. Pain 1992;48(1):5–12.

15. Rocco AG, Frank E, Kaul AF, et al. Epidural steroids, epidural morphine and epidural steroids combined with morphine in the treatment of post-laminectomy syndrome. Pain 1989;36(3):297–303.

16. Aldrete JA. Epidural injections of indomethacin for postlaminectomy syndrome: a preliminary report. Anesth Analg 2003;96(2):463–8 table of contents.

17. Aldrete JA. Recurrent neurological symptoms in a patient after repeat combined spinal and epidural anaesthesia. Br J Anaesth 2003;90(3):402–4 [author reply: 403–4].

18. Takada MF, Fukusaki M, Terrao Y, et al. Comparative efficacy of ropivacaine and bupivacaine for epidural block in outpatients with degenerative spinal disease and low back pain. Pain Clin 2005;17(3):275–81.

19. Lierz P, Gustorff B, Markow G, et al. Comparison between bupivacaine 0.125% and ropivacaine 0.2% for epidural administration to outpatients with chronic low back pain. Eur J Anaesthesiol 2004;21(1):32–7.

20. Lilius G, Harilainen A, Laasonen EM, et al. Chronic unilateral low-back pain. Predictors of outcome of facet joint injections. Spine (Phila Pa 1976) 1990;15(8):780–2.

21. Carette S, Marcoux S, Truchon R, et al. A controlled trial of corticosteroid injections into facet joints for chronic low back pain. N Engl J Med 1991;325(14):1002–7.

22. Mayer TG, Gatchel RJ, Keeley J, et al. A randomized clinical trial of treatment for lumbar segmental rigidity. Spine (Phila Pa 1976) 2004;29(20):2199–205 [discussion: 2206].

23. Marks RC, Houston T, Thulbourne T. Facet joint injection and facet nerve block: a randomised comparison in 86 patients with chronic low back pain. Pain 1992;49(3):325–8.

24. Manchikanti L, Singh V, Datta S, et al, American Society of Interventional Pain Physicians. Comprehensive review of epidemiology, scope, and impact of spinal pain. Pain Physician 2009;12(4):E35–70.

25. Fuchs S, Erbe T, Fischer HL, et al. Intraarticular hyaluronic acid versus glucocorticoid injections for nonradicular pain in the lumbar spine. J Vasc Interv Radiol 2005;16(11):1493–8.

26. Baxter GD, Bell AJ, Allen JM, et al. Low-level laser therapy: current clinical practice in Northern Ireland. Physiotherapy 1991;77:171–8.

27. Basford JR. Low-energy laser therapy: controversies and new research findings. Lasers Surg Med 1989;9(1):1–5.

28. Sakurai Y, Yamaguchi M, Abiko Y. Inhibitory effect of low-level laser irradiation on LPS-stimulated prostaglandin E2 production and cyclooxygenase-2 in human gingival fibroblasts. Eur J Oral Sci 2000;108(1):29–34.

29. Kreisler M, Christoffers AB, Al-Haj H, et al. Low level 809-nm diode laser-induced in vitro stimulation of the proliferation of human gingival fibroblasts. Lasers Surg Med 2002;30(5):365–9.
30. Saal JA, Saal JS. Intradiscal electrothermal treatment for chronic discogenic low back pain. A prospective outcome study with a minimum 2-year follow-up. Spine 2002;27:366–73.
31. Derby R, Eek B, Chen Y, et al. Intradiscal electrothermal annuloplasty (IDET): a novel approach for treating chronic discogenic back pain. Neuromodulation 2000;3(2):82–8.
32. Pauza KJ, Howell S, Dreyfuss P, et al. A randomized, placebo-controlled trial of intradiscal electrothermal therapy for the treatment of discogenic low back pain. Spine J 2004;4(1):27–35.
33. Freeman BJ, Fraser RD, Cain CM, et al. A randomized, double-blind, controlled trial: intradiscal electrothermal therapy versus placebo for the treatment of chronic discogenic low back pain. Spine (Phila Pa 1976) 2005;30(21):2369–77 [discussion: 2378].
34. Kapural L, Hayek S, Malak O, et al. Intradiscal thermal annuloplasty versus intradiscal radiofrequency ablation for the treatment of discogenic pain: a prospective matched control trial. Pain Med 2005;6(6):425–31.
35. Ercelen O, Bulutcu E, Oktenoglu T, et al. Radiofrequency lesioning using two different time modalities for the treatment of lumbar discogenic pain: a randomized trial. Spine (Phila Pa 1976) 2003;28(17):1922–7.
36. Barendse GA, van Den Berg SG, Kessels AH, et al. Randomized controlled trial of percutaneous intradiscal radiofrequency thermocoagulation for chronic discogenic back pain: lack of effect from a 90-second 70 C lesion. Spine (Phila Pa 1976) 2001;26(3):287–92.
37. Sharps LS, Isaac Z. Percutaneous disc decompression using nucleoplasty. Pain Physician 2002;5(2):121–6.
38. Masala S, Massari F, Fabiano S, et al. Nucleoplasty in the treatment of lumbar diskogenic back pain: one year follow-up. Cardiovasc Intervent Radiol 2007;30(3):426–32.
39. Singh V, Piryani C, Liao K. Role of percutaneous disc decompression using coblation in managing chronic discogenic low back pain: a prospective, observational study. Pain Physician 2004;7(4):419–25.
40. Reddy AS, Loh S, Cutts J, et al. New approach to the management of acute disc herniation. Pain Physician 2005;8(4):385–90.
41. Bhagia SM, Slipman CW, Nirschl M, et al. Side effects and complications after percutaneous disc decompression using coblation technology. Am J Phys Med Rehabil 2006;85(1):6–13.
42. Gibson JN, Grant IC, Waddell G. The Cochrane review of surgery for lumbar disc prolapse and degenerative lumbar spondylosis. Spine (Phila Pa 1976) 1999; 24(17):1820–32.
43. Nardi PV, Cabezas D, Cesaroni A. Percutaneous cervical nucleoplasty using coblation technology. Clinical results in fifty consecutive cases. Acta Neurochir Suppl 2005;92:73–8.

Surgical Treatment of Low Back Pain

Eron G. Manusov, MD

KEYWORDS

- Low back pain • Discectomy • Fusion • Low back surgery

KEY POINTS

- There is a need for quality trials that study optimal selection and timing of surgical treatment options.
- Studies need to be designed to investigate cost-effectiveness and effect on long-term improvement. Until such data are available, primary physicians should follow the guidelines published on conservative management and aggressively evaluate the red flags of low back pain, immediately refer for neurologic deficit and bowel or bladder compromise, and focus treatment on modalities with high-quality, evidence-based information.
- The 5% of patients who do not improve can be referred to surgeons with experience and expertise in discectomies. Surgical management of non–disc-disease low back pain should consider surgeons who have had success and focused surgical techniques with good outcomes.
- For those rare patients who have severe pain that has not responded to any intervention, have failed back surgery, or have complications of previous surgeries, primary care physicians should manage pain with an integrated and collaborative approach.

INTRODUCTION

This article reviews various approaches to the management of low back pain, ranging from exercise and manual or thermal techniques to invasive injections. No matter what nonsurgical approach is taken, most patients' pain either improves or resolves. However, approximately 5% of patients describe persistent low back pain despite multiple trials of rehabilitation or attempts at pain control. It is for these patients that primary care physicians must decide whether surgical intervention will make a difference. Absolute indications for surgery include progressive muscle weakness (neurologic deficit) or bowel and bladder dysfunction, but these are rare.[1,2] However, other patients may benefit from surgical intervention. This article reviews the evidence on surgical management of low back pain, which patients should be referred to surgeons, and when. It is the surgeon who chooses the procedures, but knowledge

Clinical and Educational Services, Family Medicine Residency, Duke Southern Regional AHEC, 1601 Owens Drive, Fayetteville, NC 28304, USA
E-mail address: eron.manusov@sr-ahec.org

Prim Care Clin Office Pract 39 (2012) 525–531
http://dx.doi.org/10.1016/j.pop.2012.06.010
0095-4543/12/$ – see front matter © 2012 Elsevier Inc. All rights reserved.
primarycare.theclinics.com

of high-quality study outcomes facilitates primary care physicians in making the decision of which surgeon should be consulted.

HISTORY OF SPINE SURGERY

The practice of neurosurgery did not become a specialty until the early twentieth century. However, physicians have operated on the back since antiquity. Prognosis has always been guarded and that poor prognosis applied to both the surgeon and the patient. King Hammurabi of Babylon (1955–1912 BC) outlined in his Code that:

> If a physician makes a wound and cures a freeman, he shall receive ten pieces of silver, but only five if the patient is the son of a plebeian or two if he is a slave. However, it is decreed that if a physician treats a patient with a metal knife for a severe wound and has caused the man to die—his hands shall be cut off
> —Code of Hammurabi.[3]

Early Egyptian physicians described trauma and infections of the brain and spinal cord as early as 1700 BC. It is not until the golden age of Greece, with the founding of the Alexandrian School in 300 BC, that open dissection was incorporated into formal teaching. Hippocratic writings contain numerous anatomic descriptions and reflect the early practice of spinal injuries. However, surgery on the spine was a great rarity.[3] Galen of Pergamon, who began writing at the age of 13 years and, during a career that ended with his death at age 70 years, was one of the first physicians to discuss a surgical option for the back. He was a physician at the time of Emperor Antonius Pius and Marcus Aurelius and, with experience as physician for the gladiators and his own inquisitive nature, was able to describe much of the anatomy and physiology of the spinal cord and nervous system, including the Brown-Sequard syndrome (hemisection of the cord) and Pott disease (tuberculosis of the spine). Paul of Aegineta (635–690 AD) argued that decompression (laminectomy) was in the best interest of the patient with laminar fracture and cord compression.

The Arabic schools of medicine that followed improved the practice of medicine, but because the surgery was relegated to the lower-caste surgeon and the thinking to the physician, advances in surgical technique were slow to advance. During the difficult times of the medieval period, much of medical knowledge was carefully guarded by monastic recluses; however, some surgeons, such as Theodoric of Cervia (1205–1298 AD) and William of Saliceto (1210–1277 AD) did master surgical skills that included the spine.

Wilhelm Fabricius von Hilden, also known as Guilhelmus Fabricius Hildanus, is known as the father of German Surgery and had a strong interest in pediatric and adult neurosurgery, but it was not until the early 1900s that neurosurgery became a specialty.[4,5] Harvey Williams Cushing, of Johns Hopkins University fame, is widely known as the father of modern neurosurgery. He greatly advanced the role of surgery for the treatment of low back pain.

Since the 1930s, the rate of surgery for the back has progressively increased so that the rates of back surgery in the United States are currently among the highest in the world.[1] Common surgeries for back pain include various types of fusions for nonradicular low back pain with degenerative changes, discectomy for herniation of the disc and resultant radiculopathy, and decompressive laminectomy with or without fusion for degenerative spondylolisthesis.

This article reviews the most common surgical procedures and the current evidence. Primary care physicians do not perform the surgery, but knowledge of the procedure, indication, complications, and success provides information with which to discuss possibilities with patients. Other more recent surgical procedures that include interspinous spacers, artificial discs, and various microsurgical, laser, and thermal interventions are reviewed.

SURGICAL INDICATIONS

Back surgery may be indicated for herniated lumbar disc with radiculopathy and for symptomatic spinal surgery when serious neurologic deficits are present.[1,6–8] In general, back surgery for nonradicular pain and absence of neurologic deficit, the benefits of surgery are less certain. As mentioned by Manusov elsewhere in this issue, that controversy stems from the confusing presentation of pain, difficulty in diagnosing the cause of pain, as well as research methodology flaws.

Although there have been more recent reviews and meta-analyses of specific surgical procedures that are reviewed later, the most recent Cochrane Review, published in 2007, outlines the best of all surgical interventions for lumbar disc prolapse.[9] This updated Cochran Review included evidence from 40 randomized trials and 2 quasirandomized controlled trials with a total of 5197 participants. These studies reviewed information from a surgical removal of part of the disc (discectomy), use of magnification during surgery (microdiscectomy) and injection of an enzyme into a bulging spinal disc in an effort to reduce the size of the disc (chemonucleolysis). The conclusions are that:

1. Surgical discectomy for carefully selected patients with sciatica caused by prolapsed lumbar disc can provide faster relief from pain than a nonsurgical management.
2. Long-term effects on underlying disc disease are unclear.
3. Microdiscectomy is comparable with standard discectomy.
4. There is insufficient evidence on other surgical techniques to offer conclusions, although certain surgical procedures may be appropriate if disc material is contained by the outer layers of the annulus fibrosus.
5. There are several nonsystematic reviews that compare microdiscectomy, automated percutaneous discectomy, and various types of arthroscopic microdiscectomy. The smaller incisions lead to faster patient recovery with less hospital stay time, but the long-term effect of pain and improved clinical outcomes are still questionable.

Prolapsed discs (herniated discs, ruptured discs, or herniated nucleus pulposus) are the most common cause for surgical back pain. Surgeons would like to be able to define which treatment is optimal for what type of prolapse (eg, sequestered or contained by annulus fibrosus). Study results from nonsystematic reviews published from 1995 to 2003 indicate that smaller wounds promote faster patient recovery and earlier hospital discharge. However, it is not clear whether that translates to better long-term clinical outcomes.[10–12]

The effects of interventions are summarized in the following sections. The data are reported from studies or systematic reviews that meet Cochrane Review standards.

DISCECTOMY

Surgical discectomy was compared with some form of watch and wait, conservative treatment, or placebo in 4 trials. Discectomy was significantly better than conservative therapy at 1 year, but there were no significant differences in outcomes at 4 and 10 years. Impaired motor function had better outcomes with surgery than impaired surgery than discectomy without impaired motor function.[2]

A multicenter US Spine Patient Outcomes Research Trial was published by Weinstein and colleagues[13] in 2006. This study compared standard open discectomy with nonoperative individualized treatment. The results favored surgery but there are multiple methodological challenges that make a definitive conclusion difficult. In a study that compared results following microdiscectomy with epidural steroid injection, those patients who underwent surgery had faster reduction of symptoms.

There have been at least 9 trials that compared various types of surgical procedures. In trials that compared microdiscectomy, the use of a microscope increased the surgical time but did not affect the length of hospital stay, complications, or scar formation.[14–16] There is evidence that videoarthroscopy may be useful, although no definitive data have been reported. One trial compared early outcomes and recurrence rates after sequestrectomy and microdiscectomy. The more invasive removal of disc and herniated material resulted in poorer results than sequestrectomy alone.[17]

Automated percutaneous discectomy may be inferior and suitable only for small herniations localized in front of the intervertebral space and without a tear of the posterior longitudinal ligament.[18–20] No trial has studied transforaminal endoscopic discectomy or foraminotomy. Gibson and Waddell[2] included 2 trials of laser discectomy that resulted in shrinkage of disc tissue, but no outcomes data were published.

To date, there is such heterogeneity between trial data and methodology that it is difficult to reach a conclusion about discectomy. In a specific group of patients with sciatica or neurologic deficit that corresponded with disc material compromising nerve function, who failed conservative therapy, some form of discectomy may be helpful. Results from laser microdissection vary according to the skill and experience of the surgeon. Until there is better scientific evidence, automated percutaneous discectomy, coblation therapy, and laser discectomy are considered experimental.

NONDISCECTOMY SURGERY FOR LOW BACK PAIN

Surgical procedures for low back pain that does not involve prolapsed disc material are even more controversial. The controversy surrounds both the complex nature of pain related to degeneration, subluxations, spondylolisthesis, and stenosis and the poor quality of surgical prospective, randomized controlled trials. Pain produced by processes other than prolapsed discs is variable. Therefore, the study methodology has to be concise with functional data (strength, range of motion, neurologic deficit), outcomes data (return to work, improved pain, short term vs long term) and data for comparisons with a gold standard, placebo, or standardized conservative therapy. The outcome must be chosen), the demographics must be similar), and choices must be made for the definition, a valid and reliable tool, the duration of the study, and how to control for surgical skill.

In 2008, Ibrahim and colleagues[21] pooled mean differences in the Oswestry Disability Index for 634 patients and, although there were minimal differences that favored surgical fusion, the differences were not statistically significant. The investigators advised that surgeons should cautiously recommend spinal fusion for chronic low back pain. Surgery for radiculopathy with herniated lumbar disc and symptomatic spinal stenosis is associated with short-term benefits compared with nonsurgical therapy.[1] For nonradicular low back pain associated with degeneration, fusion is no more effective than conservative therapy.

In 2011, Wood and colleagues[22] evaluated the effectiveness of spinal fusion versus structured rehabilitation in patients with chronic low back pain with and without isthmic spondylolisthesis, which is a specific subset of patients, and they included 3 randomized controlled trials that compared fusion with supervised nonoperative care in patients with chronic low back pain without isthmic spondylolisthesis; 1 randomized controlled trial evaluated these treatments in patients with isthmic spondylolisthesis. As with meta-analysis and research on back pain, there were considerable differences in type of fusion, nature of rehabilitation, patient characteristics, length of follow-up, and outcomes. The results favored surgery in patients without isthmic spondylolisthesis compared with rehabilitation. The conclusion is that fusion should be considered for patients with low back pain and isthmic spondylolisthesis who have failed nonoperative treatment.

Zhou and colleagues[23] recently published a meta-analysis of instrumented posterior interbody fusion versus instrumented posterolateral fusion in the lumbar spine. The analysis provided moderate-quality evidence that instrumented posterior lumbar interbody fusion (iPLIF) has the advantages of higher fusion rate and better restoration of spinal alignment than instrumented posterolateral fusion (iPLF) caused by degenerative lumbar disease. No significant differences were identified between iPLIF and iPLF concerning clinical outcome, complication rate, operating time, and blood loss.

DISC REPLACEMENT SURGERY

Total disc replacement is the most recent alternative to lumbar fusion. There are numerous prosthesis and trials, but, to date, there is no evidence that total disc replacement is superior to fusion. The Charite trial studied the Charite artificial disc and this was found not to be inferior to the BAK Interbody Fusion system, but there were no statistically significant differences in mean pain and physical function scores. The Prodisc artificial disc was statistically significantly more effective compared with lumbar circumferential fusion, but the risk of bias was high. Long-term benefits to total disc replacement are unknown. Well-designed prospective randomized controlled trails are needed to determine whether total disc replacement will reduce pain, improve function, and serve as an alternative to fusion.[24,25]

SUMMARY

There is still a need for quality trials that study optimal selection and timing of surgical treatment options. Studies are needed of cost-effectiveness and effect on long-term improvement. Until data from such studies are available, primary physicians should follow the guidelines on conservative management and aggressively evaluate the red flags of low back pain, immediately refer for neurologic deficit and bowel or bladder compromise, and focus treatment on modalities with high-quality evidence-based information. The 5% of patients who do not improve can be referred to surgeons with experience and expertise in discectomies. Surgical management of non–disc-disease low back pain should consider surgeons who have had success and have focused surgical techniques with good outcomes. For those rare patients who have severe pain that has not responded to any intervention, or have failed back surgery, or have complications of previous surgeries, primary care physicians should manage pain with an integrated collaborative approach to the management of pain. Future high-quality studies may improve the surgical options, but, until then, advice from our mentor, Hippocrates, should be considered: "First do no harm."

REFERENCES

1. Chou R, Baisden J, Carragee EJ, et al. Surgery for low back pain: a review of the evidence for an American Pain Society Clinical Practice Guideline. Spine 2009; 34:1094–109.

2. Gibson JN, Waddell G. Surgical interventions for lumbar disc prolapse: updated Cochrane Review. Spine 2007;32:1735–47.
3. Goodrich JT. History of spine surgery in the ancient and medieval worlds. Neurosurg Focus 2004;16:E2.
4. Dmetrichuk JM, Pendleton C, Jallo GI, et al. Father of neurosurgery: Harvey Cushing's early experience with a pediatric brainstem glioma at the Johns Hopkins Hospital. J Neurosurg Pediatr 2011;8:337–41.
5. Tubbs RS, Song YB, Loukas M, et al. Wilhelm Fabricius von Hilden (Guilhelmus Fabricius Hildanus) 1560-1634: pioneer of early neurosurgery. Childs Nerv Syst 2012;28:657–9.
6. Chou R, Atlas SJ, Stanos SP, et al. Nonsurgical interventional therapies for low back pain: a review of the evidence for an American Pain Society clinical practice guideline. Spine 2009;34:1078–93.
7. Chou R, Loeser JD, Owens DK, et al. Interventional therapies, surgery, and interdisciplinary rehabilitation for low back pain: an evidence-based clinical practice guideline from the American Pain Society. Spine 2009;34:1066–77.
8. Hayden JA, Chou R, Hogg-Johnson S, et al. Systematic reviews of low back pain prognosis had variable methods and results: guidance for future prognosis reviews. J Clin Epidemiol 2009;62:781–796.e1.
9. A trial station for integrated medicine. Hospitalis 1952;22:390–1.
10. Kahanovitz N, Viola K, Muculloch J. Limited surgical discectomy and microdiscectomy. A clinical comparison. Spine 1989;14:79–81.
11. Onik G, Mooney V, Maroon JC, et al. Automated percutaneous discectomy: a prospective multi-institutional study. Neurosurgery 1990;26:228–32 [discussion: 32–3].
12. Kambin P, NASS. Arthroscopic microdiscectomy. Spine J 2003;3:60S–4S.
13. Weinstein JN, Lurie JD, Tosteson TD, et al. Surgical vs nonoperative treatment for lumbar disk herniation: the Spine Patient Outcomes Research Trial (SPORT) observational cohort. JAMA 2006;296:2451–9.
14. Tullberg T, Isacson J, Weidenhielm L. Does microscopic removal of lumbar disc herniation lead to better results than the standard procedure? Results of a one-year randomized study. Spine 1993;18:24–7.
15. Lagarrigue J, Chaynes P. Comparative study of disk surgery with or without microscopy. A prospective study of 80 cases. Neurochirurgie 1994;40:116–20 [in French].
16. Brunon J, Chazal J, Chirossel JP, et al. When is spinal fusion warranted in degenerative lumbar spinal stenosis? Rev Rhum Engl Ed 1996;63:44–50.
17. Thome C, Barth M, Scharf J, et al. Outcome after lumbar sequestrectomy compared with microdiscectomy: a prospective randomized study. J Neurosurg Spine 2005;2:271–8.
18. Chatterjee S, Foy PM, Findlay GF. Report of a controlled clinical trial comparing automated percutaneous lumbar discectomy and microdiscectomy in the treatment of contained lumbar disc herniation. Spine 1995;20:734–8.
19. Haines SJ, Jordan N, Boen JR, et al. Discectomy strategies for lumbar disc herniation: study design and implications for clinical research. J Clin Neurosci 2002;9:440–6.
20. Haines SJ, Jordan N, Boen JR, et al. Discectomy strategies for lumbar disc herniation: results of the LAPDOG trial. J Clin Neurosci 2002;9:411–7.
21. Ibrahim T, Tleyjeh IM, Gabbar O. Surgical versus non-surgical treatment of chronic low back pain: a meta-analysis of randomised trials. Int Orthop 2008;32:107–13.

22. Wood KB, Fritzell P, Dettori JR, et al. Effectiveness of spinal fusion versus structured rehabilitation in chronic low back pain patients with and without isthmic spondylolisthesis: a systematic review. Spine 2011;36:S110–9.
23. Zhi-Jie Zhou, Feng-Dong Zhao, Xiang-Qian Fang, et al. Meta-analysis of instrumented posterior interbody fusion versus instrumented posterolateral fusion in the lumbar spine: a review. J Neurosurg Spine 2011;15:295–310.
24. van den Eerenbeemt KD, Ostelo RW, van Royen BJ, et al. Total disc replacement surgery for symptomatic degenerative lumbar disc disease: a systematic review of the literature. Eur Spine J 2010;19:1262–80.
25. Freeman BJ, Davenport J. Total disc replacement in the lumbar spine: a systematic review of the literature. Eur Spine J 2006;15(Suppl 3):S439–47.

Complementary and Alternative Medicine Treatments for Low Back Pain

Dan Marlowe, PhD, LMFT

KEYWORDS

- Low back pain • Complimentary and alternative medicine • Operant therapies
- Integrative medicine

KEY POINTS

- Depending on type, behavioral treatments augment cognitions, emotions, perceptions, and/or physical responses experienced by the patient regarding the diagnosis and/or the perceived disability associated with it. Treatments of this nature can be broken down into 3 typologies: (1) operant-based, (2) cognitive-based, and (3) respondent-based therapies,[1] which are determined by the theoretic basis and aim of the modality of treatment.
- Operant therapies are typically used to replace behaviors that promote and reinforce pain associated with low back pain (LBP) with behaviors that result in increased social engagement (eg, work and family) and pain reduction (eg, hobbies and physical activity).
- Cognitive therapy for LBP entails the identification and augmentation of thoughts, patterns of thought, feelings, and beliefs that have a negative impact on the adjustment of a patient. The main goal of this therapeutic modality is the modification of a patient's experience of the diagnosis, associated disability, and/or lifestyle changes through the challenging of cognitions, feelings, and/or beliefs.
- Just as cognitive therapy seeks to challenge thoughts, feelings, and beliefs by interrupting the patterns of how they develop, respondent therapy attempts to interrupt the physiologic response of a patient to the sensation of pain.[1] This response is typified through muscle tension, which exacerbates the patient's sensation of the pain, thereby continuing and amplifying the subsequent physiologic response.
- Several studies have investigated the effectiveness of acupuncture compared with no treatment or sham treatment, comparative studies between acupuncture and other interventions, as well as studies investigating the addition of acupuncture as an adjunctive interventional strategy. Compared with no treatment, acupuncture was effective for short-term and medium-term pain relief for patients, as well as short-term functional improvement with no difference for intermediate-term follow-up.
- Based on the effectiveness research available, neuroreflexotherapy (NRT), compared with sham NRT, achieved statistically significant pain reduction at both 30-day and 45-day follow-ups, with patients in the NRT group reporting major relief or pain disappearance.[2,3]

Department of Applied Psychosocial Medicine, Southern Regional Area Health Education Center, 1601 Owen Drive, Fayetteville, NC 28304, USA
E-mail address: daniel.marlowe@sr-ahec.org

Prim Care Clin Office Pract 39 (2012) 533–546
http://dx.doi.org/10.1016/j.pop.2012.06.008
0095-4543/12/$ – see front matter
© 2012 Elsevier Inc. All rights reserved.

COMPLEMENTARY AND ALTERNATIVE MEDICINE, INTEGRATIVE MEDICINE, AND LOW BACK PAIN

Given the large number of the general population who have low back pain (LBP; there is a lifetime prevalence of 65%–80% in the United States),[4] as well as the ambiguous pathophysiology of the condition,[5] many patients often seek out complimentary and alternative medicine (CAM) in an adjunctive capacity with contemporary treatment (**Figs. 1** and **2**). This article presents 6 such therapies (ie, behavioral treatment, acupuncture, manipulation, prolotherapy, neuroreflexotherapy, and herbal treatments), which are discussed in terms of the specifics of the modality, as well as the empirical evidence related to its effectiveness.

Behavioral Treatment

Regardless of the severity of the condition, patients who experience chronic LBP often find that they must change their lifestyle and activity level to better accommodate the physical impacts (eg, pain) of the diagnosis.[5] Adjustment in this context does not only mean the way in which they engage in physical activity, but their thoughts, emotions, and experience of the diagnosis, associated pain, and lifestyle changes. Depending on many different interpersonal and intrapersonal factors (eg, severity of condition, individual pain threshold, social support, degree of lifestyle change required), how patients go about adjusting, and the degree to which they do so often affects their ability to manage the condition both biologically and psychosocially.[6,7] From a practical standpoint, a patient who does not adjust well to LBP, or any other medical condition, may develop depressive and/or anxious conditions that affect and further exacerbate the associated pain. Depending on how these comorbid psychosocial diagnoses develop in relation to the biologic condition, patients most notably may experience increased muscle tension and social withdrawal,[1] both of which can intensify their experience of the pain, further hindering their adjustment.

Behavioral treatments, depending on type, augment cognitions, emotions, perceptions, and/or physical responses experienced by the patient regarding the diagnosis and/or the perceived disability associated with it. Treatments of this nature can be

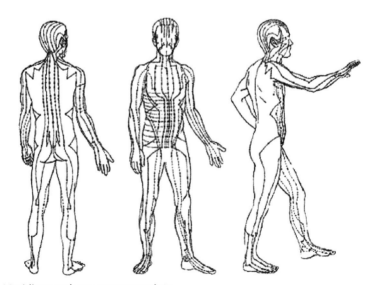

Fig. 1. Meridians and acupuncture points.

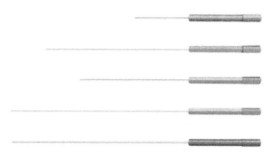

Fig. 2. Acupuncture needle sizes.

broken down into 3 typologies: (1) operant-based, (2) cognitive-based, and (3) respondent-based therapies,[1] which are determined by the theoretic basis and aim of the modality of treatment. (**Box 1**) These therapies are rarely, if ever, used alone, but instead are used in conjunction with one another. Patients who are diagnosed with LBP and are experiencing significant difficulty with adjustment may have regular psychotherapy to deal with their thoughts about the diagnosis (ie, cognitive therapy), negotiate with their providers a schedule for engaging in physical activity a certain number of times in a week (eg, operant therapy), as well as learn progressive muscle relaxation for use when there is breakthrough pain (ie, respondent therapy).

Operant Therapy

Operant therapies are typically used to replace behaviors that promote and reinforce pain associated with LBP with behaviors that result in increased social engagement (eg, work and family) and pain reduction (eg, hobbies and physical activity). From this perspective, patients who have LBP often find external reinforcement for those behaviors associated with the pain itself (eg, attention from family members and the medical community, use of medication to reduce level of pain).[8] In order to replace these behaviors with those preferable for pain reduction, the use of concrete goal setting and the formation of behavioral quotas are often used. An acronym for goal setting, SMART (specific, measurable, attainable, realistic, and time bound), is 1 way to ensure that patients and their loved ones are able to be successful in achieving these goals.[9] Once an SMART goal is set, the nature of the accompanying quota is

---

Box 1
Types of behavioral therapy

Operant therapy

Replaces unwanted behaviors with preferred behaviors through the setting and reinforcement of behavioral quotas (eg, walk 1 km twice a week).

Cognitive therapy

Helps patients identify and replace unwanted patterns of thoughts, beliefs, and/or perceptions through a combination of distraction and thought-stopping techniques (eg, when a patient thinks "I am hopeless" they recognize the thought and then focus on things in their life that are positive: eg, family, friends, children).

Respondant therapy

Helps patients modulate their experience of pain (ie, muscle tension) through changing their physiologic response to unpleasant stimuli using relaxation techniques (eg, progressive relaxation).

typically individualized (eg, a patient who has LBP and is obese may only be able to walk 1 km once a week instead of 3 times a week), but usually revolves around exercise, social engagement, or both. Patients are expected to meet the quota on a predetermined timeline, with the quota then being increased after each completion point is successfully achieved. Significant others, family members, and friends are often recruited to help with reinforcing these behaviors because positive reinforcement is given to the patient by family, friends, and treatment staff throughout the attempt and every time a quota is successfully met.

Cognitive Therapy

Cognitive therapy for LBP entails the identification and augmentation of thoughts, patterns of thought, feelings, and beliefs that have a negative impact on the adjustment of a patient. The main goal of this therapeutic modality is the modification of a patient's experience of the diagnosis, associated disability, and/or lifestyle changes through the challenging of cognitions, feelings, and/or beliefs. How patients perceive their pain, as well as the degree to which they perceive their locus of control over it (ie, internal or external), plays a large role in their experience and overall management of the condition.[6,7] Challenging patients' perception of pain and their ability to manage it is typically done through multiple modalities (eg, health education, psychoeducation, psychotherapy), as well as the use of techniques designed to stop thoughts and/or redirect their focus.[10] At first, patients are often asked to keep a diary or some type of log of their thoughts over the course of a period of time to better understand and uncover possible triggers and patterns. Once identified, these patterns can be interrupted by the thought-stopping and/or redirecting techniques mentioned earlier, or through the use of a combination of other types of intervention (quotas, exercise programs, and so forth).[6]

Respondent Therapy

Just as cognitive therapy seeks to challenge thoughts, feelings, and beliefs by interrupting the patterns of how they develop, respondent therapy attempts to interrupt the physiologic response of a patient to the sensation of pain.[1] This response is typified through muscle tension, which exacerbates the patient's sensation of the pain, thereby continuing and amplifying the subsequent physiologic response. Respondent therapies like biofeedback and progressive muscle relaxation allow patients to interrupt this pain-tension cycle by introducing relaxation techniques into the sequence. The introduction of these techniques at key points within the cycle allows the patient to deescalate the process, thereby improving both their tension and subsequent pain. Many types of biofeedback exist; however, the electromyogram (EMG) is primarily used to help patients with this muscular tension.[1] This technique involves the placement of EMG sensors on the body in areas that experience significant tension during the pain-tension cycle. During the cycle, the sensors visually register this tension on a computer screen, and patients can then attempt to modulate their response. An example of this type of visual modulation would be a sad face that gradually turns into a happy face as the patient relaxes the muscles in the affected area. Progressive muscle relaxation functions in a similar capacity, in that a patient actively tenses and relax muscles over a short period of time. Patients are typically asked to tense muscles in certain parts of the body for 10 seconds then relaxing for 20 seconds, with a session lasting up to 30 minutes.[11]

Empirical Support

Multiple studies have investigated the clinical effectiveness of behavioral interventions compared with wait list controls (ie, groups that are not provided the treatment for a period of time), the comparison of different types of behavioral treatments, and there are 2 Cochrane Reviews dedicated to the subject.[12–14] Operant therapy alone was more effective than wait list for reduction of pain in the short term; however, it did not have a significant impact on either improved functional status or depressive symptoms compared with wait list controls[15,16] (evidence level B, lower quality randomized controlled trial [RCT]). Cognitive therapy by itself did not produce a significant difference for patients for either pain reduction or functional status compared with wait list controls[10,17] (evidence level A, RCT; evidence level B, lower quality RCT). For respondent therapies, there is evidence to support reduced pain for patients compared with wait list controls, as well as evidence supporting improved functional status for patients using progressive muscle relaxation but not biofeedback.[10,18–21] However, both typologies of respondent therapy showed no significant difference compared with wait list controls for depressive symptoms. Combined typologies of behavioral intervention were effective compared with wait list controls for pain reduction, but showed no significant difference for patients on functional status and depressive symptoms.[10,16,18,21,22]

In terms of comparison studies, EGM biofeedback was more effective than progressive muscle relaxation in both the short and intermediate terms for pain reduction[23] (evidence level B, lower quality RCT); however, no significant difference was found when respondent therapy was compared with cognitive therapy.[10] There were similar findings when cognitive therapy was also compared with operant therapy.[24,25] Several studies comparing behavioral therapies alone with combined behavioral interventions found no significant differences on pain reduction, functional status, or depressive symptoms.[10,16,18,21,25–27]

ACUPUNCTURE

The philosophic underpinnings of acupuncture come from Chinese philosophy related to the flow of life force or energy (Qi; pronounced chi) throughout the body.[28] This energy, which flows through channels within the body called meridians, exists in a state of balance between dark (Yin) and light (Yang) properties. In terms of this philosophic orientation, disease manifests when Qi becomes unbalanced and its flow obstructed through the meridians, which leads to further unbalancing and progression of the disease state.[28] Because of the close proximity of meridians and Qi to the surface of the skin, the placement of needles on specific points, of which there 361, along these meridians is thought to help rebalance the proportion of Yin and Yang aspects of Qi by helping to facilitate its flow throughout the body.

Needles

Acupuncture needles have been made out of numerous materials including ceramic, bamboo, bronze, iron, and gold, with modern needles constructed of stainless steel.[28] Typically needles are composed of 5 parts: (1) handle, (2) tail, (3) tip, (4) body, and (5) root, and diameters range from 0.2 to 0.28 mm, whereas length can range from 15 to 60 mm.[28] During the manufacturing process, needles are sterilized with either ethylene oxide gas or radiation, and are packaged together in microbial barrier packaging paper. Packaging of needles is required to meet US Food and Drug Administration standards, which includes the name of the product and manufacturer, lot number, size and number of the needles, packaging process, storage conditions, method and date of sterilization, and date of expiration.[28]

Technique

Although acupuncture in the classical sense has existed in the Western world for several hundred years, and in Eastern countries for several thousand, modifications to this technique has yielded different permutations of needle placement, as well as augmentations to their stimulation. Although all permutations are based on traditional Chinese philosophy and medical practice, there has been the development of differing schools of acupuncture within the last several decades, as well as the development of different forms of the practice (eg, auricular, scalp, nose, and foot).[28] Once needles are placed in the body, they are angled to the skin at 90, 45, or 15° based on the location of the acupuncture point, the purpose of the session, and the patient's size.[28] After insertion, the needles are usually manipulated by the practitioner to stimulate the body's healing response by lifting and thrusting, twirling and rotating, or a combination; however, in certain practices, modern elements have been added to the needles to amplify their effect. Modern additives to acupuncture needles include electroacupuncture (in which an electrical current is added to the needle after insertion), injection acupuncture (in which herbals tinctures are injected into the site), laser acupuncture, and magnetic acupuncture. Through manipulation, practitioners feel for tenseness around the needle, which signifies the patient's experience of De Qi, which is a sensation of heaviness, numbness, and/or tightness.[28]

Empirical Support

Several studies have investigated the effectiveness of acupuncture compared with no treatment or sham treatment, comparing acupuncture with other interventions, as well as studies investigating the addition of acupuncture as an adjunctive interventional strategy. Compared with no treatment, acupuncture was effective for short-term and medium-term pain relief for patients, as well as short-term functional improvement, with no difference for intermediate-term follow-up evidence level B, lower quality RCT).[29,30] Compared with sham therapy, several studies found a significant difference for patients regarding pain relief immediately following the acupuncture session, along with evidence to imply that the analgesic effects are also apparent at both intermediate-term and long-term follow-up (Refs.[30,31,33,34] evidence level B, lower quality RCT; Refs.[29,31] evidence level A, RCT].[31–36]

Compared with pharmacologic modalities, no difference in short-term pain relief or functionality was found between acupuncture and naproxen, celecoxib, rofecoxib, or paracetamol.[37,38] Also, no differences in pain relief and functionally were noted for acupuncture compared with self-care education and massage, and acupuncture was less effective than spinal manipulation.[37,39] Comparative studies for acupuncture as an adjunctive treatment to other interventions (ie, exercise, nonsteroidal antiinflammatory drugs [NSAIDs], aspirin, nonnarcotic analgesic, mud packs, infrared heat therapy, back care education, ergonomics, and/or behavioral modification) against other interventions alone, shows significant pain reduction immediately following the intervention, as well as at both short-term and intermediate-term follow-up.[34,36,40,41]

MANIPULATION

Used in some form for more than 2000 years, spinal manipulative therapy (SMT) involves the use of high-impact-velocity impulse or thrust at the synovial joint at or near the end of the physiologic range of motion.[42] During manipulation, the clinician controls the velocity, magnitude, and direction of the impulse. This motion subsequently causes cavitation within the fluid, which is the creation of fluid-free areas or bubbles and is achieved through the reduction of pressure within the joint itself. The formation and activity of these bubbles accounts for the audible cracking or popping sound that is characteristic of this type of therapy and is an indication of the proper application of the technique.[42,43] In contrast, mobilization uses low-grade velocity and passive movement that remains within the patient's range of motion and control to achieve a similar effect.[44] Many different health professionals use some form of manipulative therapy in their practice (eg, osteopaths, allopaths trained in manipulation, chiropractors); however, the focus and reasoning behind the application of the technique may differ based on professional affiliation.[45]

Mechanism of Action

Although several hypotheses have been proposed for the mode of action for SMT, 2 organizing categories exist: (1) mechanical, and (2) neurophysiologic.[43,44] However, a common theme of all theories is that changes to the anatomic, physiologic, or biomechanical functioning of spinal vertebrae can have negative impacts on the nervous system. From the mechanical perspective, manipulation of the functional spinal lesion (or subluxation) relieves mechanical stress at the site, which in turn leads to decreased symptom presentation.[44] This decrease is thought to be a consequence of the effect of manipulation on the inflow of information to the body's central nervous system. Neurophysiologic explanations tend to center on manipulation's impact on the motor control system, afferent neurons in paraspinal tissues, overall pain processing, and outflow of information to the autonomic nervous system, although the mode of action remains unclear.[43]

Empirical Support

Multiple studies have examined the effect of SMT compared with sham therapies, other interventions for LBP, as well as comparisons between the use of SMT as an adjunctive therapy and the primary intervention alone. Compared with sham SMT, no significant difference was found in pain reduction at 3 and 6 months, as well as no significant difference in functional status at 1, 3, or 6 months.[46–48] However, compared with all other interventions for LBP, SMT produced statistically significant greater pain reduction at 1 and 6 months, but those differences were not apparent at 12-month follow-up.[49–62]

In terms of functional status, SMT produced greater statistically significant improvement at 1 month, but no difference compared with other interventions at 3, 6, or 12 months.[49–62] Studies in which a combination of a primary therapy and SMT as an adjunctive were compared with the primary intervention alone found that combined SMT therapy had statistically significant pain reduction at 1, 3, and 12 months, but no difference in pain reduction at 6 months.[47,55,63] For functional status, SMT combined therapy achieved statistically significant improvement at 1, 3, and 12 months, but failed to yield statistical significance at 6 months compared with the primary therapy by itself[47,55,64] (Refs.[45,53] evidence level A, RCT; Ref.[62] evidence level B, lower quality RCT).

PROLOTHERAPY

Prolotherapy involves the injection of various types of solutions into damaged joints, which in turn facilitates the body's healing process through inflammation of the connective tissue. In theory, musculoskeletal pain is caused by inadequate strength and repair of stretched or torn ligaments and tendons caused by both biologic (eg, poor blood flow to the affected area) and biobehavioral impacts (eg, smoking, sleep deprivation, vitamin deficiency).[65] Once these tissues are damaged, any load-bearing activity causes the stimulation of pain mechanoreceptors that continue to be stimulated with use. Lack of adequate repair to these connective tissues leads to tissue, and ultimately joint, instability, with musculoskeletal pain being the eventual consequence.[65]

Through the injection of various solutions directly into the joint, inflammation occurs that causes granulocytes, macrophages, and fibroblasts to be drawn to the site along with the secretion of growth factors in the affected tissues. It is this process of inflammation that starts or restarts the repair and growth of these ligaments and/or tendons, thereby increasing tissue and joint stability and causing decreased pain.[66,67] In terms of chronic LBP, although typically thought to originate from herniated discs, the argument for this therapy is that disc herniations are preceded by weak spinal ligaments.[65] The laxity of the ligament provides the room necessary for the disc to herniate through it, and, even after the acute episode subsides, the 10% of patients who continue to experience chronic LBP do so because of a lack of support by the connective tissue surrounding the disc, and they face heightened odds of further injury. In addition, the weakening of the ligament and the subsequent change in biomechanics can cause the joint to become osteoarthritic, along with placing increased stress on surrounding joints.[65]

Solutions

Three primary types of solutions are used in prolotherapy: (1) irritant, (2) chemotactic, and (3) osmotic solutions.[66] Irritant solutions include phenol, guaiacol, tannic acid, and pumic flour (a type of irritant solution known as a particulate). The introduction of these solutions into the joint causes direct cellular trauma and inflammation of the tissue, which attracts macrophages and other reparative cells; chemotactic solutions operate in a similar capacity and are made from sodium morrhuate.[66] Osmotic solutions are typically composed of phenol, glycerin, and dextrose, and cause a higher of degree of inflammation of the tissue than the previous 2 categories of solution. Hypertonic dextrose is most commonly used, with a range of 12.5% to 25% (15% is the most common), and, because of the pain associated with the injection, lidocaine or another local anesthetic is typically added to the solution.[65]

Empirical Support

Several studies have examined the efficacy of prolotherapy on scores related to pain and disability compared with control injections alone, as well as when prolotherapy was used as an adjunctive to another therapy and compared with control injections. Prolotherapy alone did not produce statistically significant reductions in pain scores at 6 months compared with control injections,[68–70] but 2 studies did report statistically significant pain reduction for the treatment group when prolotherapy was used in an adjunctive capacity.[71,72] In terms of disability scores, prolotherapy alone did not produce a statistically significant difference for respondents in the treatment group; however, as with the studies comparing pain scores, prolotherapy produced a statistically significant difference for the treatment group when used in combination with another therapeutic modality (eg, spinal manipulation therapy, exercise)[70–72] (evidence level B, lower quality RCT; evidence level C, expert opinion; evidence level B, lower quality RCT).

NEUROREFLEXOTHERAPY

A new treatment of LBP, neuroreflexotherapy (NRT) involves the implantation of several epidermal staples, as well as subcutaneously implanted burins (small metallic punches) on specific dermatomes along the back with concurrent implantation of staples at referred tender points in the ear.[73,74] These devices are normally implanted at a superficial depth of less than 2 mm, and typically last up to 90 days in the back and 20 days in the ear before being removed; the burins fall out on their own after

14 days.[74] The procedure for implantation is performed on an outpatient basis, is typically completed within 60 minutes, and there has been no reported pain or scarring associated with the procedure.[74]

The mode of action for NRT centers on inhibition of 3 neural processes that make up the pathophysiology of LBP: (1) neurons responsible for perception, transmission, and integration of pain; (2) neurons related to the maintenance of muscular contraction; and (3) neurons related to neurogenic inflammation.[73,74] Stimulation of the dermatomes associated with the dermal nerve endings promotes the release of enkephalins, which bind to and inhibit the activation of nociceptive neurons, thereby inhibiting the outflow of pain signals.[74] Implantation of staples at points within the ear are thought to stimulate structures in both the thalamus and brain stem that trigger pain-relieving effects as well, which are thought to result from the connection of the ear's innervation-related nuclei.[73] Although often compared with acupuncture, NRT differs in several distinct ways: (1) theoretic basis for the therapy, (2) zones of the skin chosen for stimulation are based on their innervations and not proximity to meridians, and (3) the method of stimulation.

Empirical Support

Based on the effectiveness research available, NRT, compared with sham NRT, achieved statistically significant pain reduction at both 30-day and 45-day follow-ups, with patients in the NRT group reporting major relief or pain disappearance.[2,3] The size of pain reduction for patients in the NRT group was 60% immediately following the intervention and 50% when measured again 45 days later, as opposed to the control group whose pain reduction immediately following the intervention and 45 days later were 20% and 10%, respectively.[3] NRT also substantially improved the ability of patients to perform daily activities, with 88% of patients reporting improvement, as opposed to the 3% of patients in the control group.[2] The same 1993 study also showed improvement in the functional ability of patients receiving NRT, as shown by 96% of those patients showing improvement and only 3% showing similar improvement in the control group.

Compared with standard care, NRT produced greater reduction in pain severity, as well as statistically significant greater improvement in disability at the end of a follow-up period of 60 days.[73] However, NRT did not show greater statistically significant improvement to quality of life, although both experimental and control groups did report improvement.

HERBAL MEDICINE

Although many different categories of herbal medicine are purported to have biochemical properties that improve pain, several have been specifically tested for use with LBP (ie, *Harpagophytum procumbens, Salix alba, Capsicum frutescens*). Regarding the modes of action for these herbs in particular: (1) *C frutescens* is thought to deplete substance P (ie, neuropeptide associated with inflammatory processes and pain), (2) *H procumbens* acts as an antiinflammatory and analgesic, and (3) *S alba* is also considered an analgesic.[75,76] Use of these extracts typically involves the direct ingestion of the substance, creation of salves or gels that are applied to the affected area, or the creation of casts in which the extract is a part of the plaster.

Empirical Support

H procumbens (Devil's claw)
Several studies have compared the effectiveness of this extract with placebo, as well as its effectiveness at different doses (50 mg and 100 mg). Compared with placebo, at

the 50-mg dose, the extract increased the number of patients reporting mild to no LBP over the course of 4 weeks from 1% to 24%, as well as decreasing the number of patients complaining of severe pain: 59% at week 1 and 35% at week 4.[76,77] With the higher dose, patients reported the absence of pain for at least 5 days during the fourth week of treatment, which was not found at the lower 50 mg dosage. Although the rate of tramadol usage to help control the pain decreased for patients receiving the 50-mg dose, it did not reach statistical significance, meaning that the effect for patients was negligible. Also, in a study that compared the extract (at 60 mg per day) with rofecoxib (at 12.5 mg per day), there was no statistically significant difference in the number of patients who reported at least 5 pain-free days during the sixth week of the protocol.[78]

S alba (white willow)

When compared with placebo, both 120-mg and 240-mg doses of salicin produced statistically significant increases in the number patients reporting pain-free days during the fourth week of the protocol: placebo group, N = 4; 120-mg group, N = 15; 240-mg group, N = 27.[79,80] In another study that compared a daily dosage of 240 mg of salicin with 12.5 mg of rofecoxib, there was no statistical difference between the groups, with both reporting a 44% improvement on pain and physical disability indexes.[81] In addition, patients who needed to take adjunctive medication for breakthrough pain (NSAIDs, tramadol, or both) while following the protocol was 10% for the salicin group and 13% for the rofecoxib group,[81] which implies that the herbal preparation alone was adequate in terms of pain control for most of the experimental group.

C frutescens (species of chili pepper)

Several studies have shown that a capsicum gel, as well as a plaster cast, produces statistically significant improvements in pain scores and physical disability compared with placebo.[75,82,83] Specifically for the capsicum plaster, at least a 30% reduction in pain was reported by 60.9% of the patients compared with the 42.1% of patients reporting similar decreases in the placebo group.[75] This finding was also similar to the improvement in physical disability, with 21% of patients in the capsicum group reporting improvement compared with only 10% of patients in the placebo group. Similar findings were also echoed in a study comparing the effects of a capsicum-based gel with that of a homeopathic gel, in which both groups reported significant reductions in pain, but there was no statistically significant difference between the 2 groups in the reduction in pain scores.[84]

REFERENCES

1. Vlaeyen JWS, Haazen IWC, Schuerman JA, et al. Behavioural rehabilitation of chronic low back pain: comparison of an operant treatment, an operant cognitive treatment and an operant-respondent treatment. Br J Clin Psychol 1995;34: 95–118.
2. Kovacs FM, Abraira V, López-Abente G, et al. Neuroreflexotherapy intervention in the treatment of nonspecific low back pain: a randomized, double-blind, controlled clinical trial. [La intervención neurorreflejoterápica en el tratamiento de la lumbalgia inespecífica: un ensayo clinic controlado, aleatorizado, a doble ciego]. Med Clin (Barc) 1993;101:570–5 [spanish].
3. Kovacs FM, Abraira V, Pozo F, et al. Local and remote sustained trigger point therapy for exacerbations of chronic low back pain. Spine 1997;22:786–97.
4. Manchikanti L. Epidemiology of low back pain. Pain Physician 2000;3(3):167–92.

5. Waddell G. The back pain revolution. 2nd edition. London: Churchill Livingstone; 2004.
6. Pincus T, Vogel S, Burton AK, et al. Fear avoidance and prognosis in back pain: a systematic review and synthesis of current evidence. Arthritis Rheum 2006; 54(12):3999–4010.
7. Rudy TE, Turk DC. Cognitive-behavioral treatment of the patient with chronic pain. In: White AH, Schofferman JA, editors. Spine care volume 1: diagnosis and conservative treatment. St Louis (MO): Mosby-Year Book; 1995.
8. Fordyce WE. Behavioral methods for chronic pain and illness. St Louis (MO): Mosby; 1976.
9. Schut HA, Stam J. Goals in rehabilitation teamwork. Disabil Rehabil 1994;16(4): 223–6.
10. Turner JA, Jensen MP. Efficacy of cognitive therapy for chronic low back pain. Pain 1993;52:169–77.
11. Field T. Progressive muscle relaxation. Complementary and alternative therapies research. Washington, DC: American Psychological Association; 2009. p. 97–101.
12. Henschke N, Ostelo RWJG, van Tulder MW, et al. Behavioural treatment for chronic low-back pain. Cochrane Database Syst Rev 2010;(7):CD002014. http://dx.doi.org/10.1002/14651858.CD002014.pub3.
13. Ostelo RW, van Tulder MW, Vlaeyen JWS, et al. Behavioural treatment for chronic low-back pain. Cochrane Database Syst Rev 2005;(1):CD002014. http://dx.doi.org/10.1002/14651858.CD002014.pub2.
14. Linton SJ, Bradley LA, Jensen I, et al. The secondary prevention of low back pain: a controlled study with follow-up. Pain 1989;36:197–207.
15. Turner JA, Clancy S, McQuade KJ, et al. Effectiveness of behavioral therapy for chronic low back pain: a component analysis. J Consult Clin Psychol 1990;58:573–9.
16. Turner JA, Clancy S. Comparison of operant behavioral and cognitive-behavioral group treatment for chronic low back pain. J Consult Clin Psychol 1988;56:261–6.
17. Linton SJ, Boersma K, Jansson M, et al. A randomized controlled trial of exposure in vivo for patients with spinal pain reporting fear of work related activities. Eur J Pain 2008;12:722–30.
18. Newton-John TR, Spence SH, Schotte D. Cognitive behavioural therapy versus EMG biofeedback in the treatment of chronic low back pain. Behav Res Ther 1995;33:691–7.
19. Nouwen A. EMG biofeedback used to reduce standing levels of paraspinal muscle tension in chronic low back pain. Pain 1983;17:353–60.
20. Stuckey SJ, Jacobs A, Goldfarb J. EMG biofeedback training, relaxation training, and placebo for the relief of chronic back pain. Percept Mot Skills 1986;63: 1023–36.
21. Turner JA. Comparison of group progressive-relaxation training and cognitive-behavioral group therapy for chronic low back pain. J Consult Clin Psychol 1982;50:757–65.
22. Smeets RJ, Vlaeyen JW, Hidding A, et al. Active rehabilitation for chronic low back pain: cognitive behavioral, physical, or both? First direct post-treatment results from a randomized controlled trial. BMC Musculoskelet Disord 2006;7:5.
23. Donaldson S, Romney D, Donaldson M, et al. Randomized study of the application of single motor unit biofeedback training to chronic low back pain. J Occup Rehabil 1994;4:23–37.
24. Leeuw M, Goossens ME, van Breukelen GJP, et al. Exposure in vivo versus operant graded activity in chronic low back pain patients: results of a randomized controlled trial. Pain 2008;138:192–207.

25. Nicholas MK, Wilson PH, Goyen J. Operant-behavioural and cognitive behavioural treatment for chronic low back pain. Behav Res Ther 1991;29:225–38.
26. Kole-Snijders AM, Vlaeyen JW, Goossens ME. Chronic low back pain: what does cognitive coping skills training add to operant behavioral treatment? Results of a randomized clinical trial. J Consult Clin Psychol 1999;67:931–44.
27. van den Hout JH, Vlaeyen JW, Heuts PH, et al. Secondary prevention of work-related disability in nonspecific low back pain: does problem solving therapy help? Clin J Pain 2003;19(2):87–96.
28. Lao L. Acupuncture techniques and devices. J Altern Complement Med 1996; 2(1):23–5.
29. Coan RM, Wong G, Ku SL, et al. The acupuncture treatment of low back pain: a randomized controlled study. Am J Chin Med 1980;8:181–9.
30. Thomas M, Lundberg T. Importance of modes of acupuncture in the treatment of chronic nociceptive low back pain. Acta Anaesthesiol Scand 1994;38:63–9.
31. Carlsson CP, Sjolund BH. Acupuncture for chronic low back pain: a randomized placebo-controlled study with long-term follow-up. Clin J Pain 2001;17(4): 296–305.
32. Kerr DP, Walsh DM, Baxter D. Acupuncture in the management of chronic low back pain: a blinded randomized controlled trial. Clin J Pain 2003;19:364–70.
33. Lehmann TR, Russell DW, Spratt KF, et al. Efficacy of electroacupuncture and TENS in the rehabilitation of chronic low back pain patients. Pain 1986;26:277–90.
34. Leibing E, Leonhardt U, Koster G, et al. Acupuncture treatment of chronic low-back pain – a randomized, blinded, placebo-controlled trial with 9-month follow-up. Pain 2002;96(1–2):189–96.
35. Mendelson G, Selwood TS, Kranz H, et al. Acupuncture treatment of chronic back pain: a double-blind placebo-controlled trial. Am J Med 1983;74:49–55.
36. Molsberger AF, Mau J, Pawelec DB, et al. Does acupuncture improve the orthopedic management of chronic low back pain–a randomized, blinded, controlled trial with 3 months follow up. Pain 2002;99(3):579–87.
37. Giles LGF, Muller R. Chronic spinal pain. A randomized clinical trial comparing medication, acupuncture and spinal manipulation. Spine 2003;28(14):1490–503.
38. Kittang G, Melvaer T, Baerheim A. Acupuncture contra antiphlogistics in acute lumbago. Tidsskr Nor Laegeforen 2001;121(10):1207–10 [in Norwegian].
39. Cherkin DC, Eisenberg D, Sherman KJ, et al. Randomized trial comparing traditional Chinese medical acupuncture, therapeutic massage, and self-care education for chronic low back pain. Arch Intern Med 2001;161(8):1081–8.
40. Meng CF, Wang D, Ngeow J, et al. Acupuncture for chronic low back pain in older patients: a randomized, controlled trial. Rheumatology 2003;42:1–10.
41. Yeung CK, Leung MC, Chow DH. The use of electroacupuncture in conjunction with exercise for the treatment of chronic low-back pain. J Altern Complement Med 2003;9(4):479–90.
42. Evans DW. Mechanisms and effects of spinal high-velocity, low-amplitude thrust manipulation: previous theories. J Manipulative Physiol Ther 2002;25:251–62.
43. Triano JJ. Biomechanics of spinal manipulative therapy. Spine J 2001;1:121–30.
44. Pickar JG. Neurophysiological effects of spinal manipulation. Spine J 2002;2: 357–71.
45. van de Veen EA, de Vet HC, Pool JJ, et al. Variance in manual treatment of nonspecific low back pain between orthomanual physicians, manual therapists, and chiropractors. J Manipulative Physiol Ther 2005;28:108–16.
46. Ghroubi S, Elleuch H, Baklouti S, et al. Chronic low back pain and vertebral manipulation. Ann Readapt Med Phys 2007;50(7):570–6 [in French].

47. Licciardone JC, Stoll ST, Fulda KG, et al. Osteopathic manipulative treatment for chronic low back pain: a randomized controlled trial. Spine 2003;28(13):1355–62.

48. Waagen GN, Haldeman S, Cook G, et al. Short term trial of chiropractic adjustments for the relief of chronic low back pain. Man Med 1986;2:63–7.

49. Brønfort G, Goldsmith CH, Nelson CF, et al. Trunk exercises combined with spinal manipulative or NSAID therapy for chronic low back pain: a randomized, observer-blinded clinical trial. J Manipulative Physiol Ther 1996;19:570–82.

50. Ferreira ML, Ferreira PH, Latimer J, et al. Comparison of general exercise, motor control exercise and spinal manipulative therapy for chronic low back pain: a randomized trial. Pain 2007;131:31–7.

51. Gibson T, Grahame R, Harkness J, et al. Controlled comparison of short-wave diathermy treatment with osteopathic treatment in non-specific low back pain. Lancet 1985;8440:1258–61.

52. Gudavalli MR, Cambron JA, McGregor M, et al. A randomized clinical trial and subgroup analysis to compare flexion-distraction with active exercise for chronic low back pain. Eur Spine J 2006;15(7):1070–82.

53. Hemmila HM, Keinanen-Kiukaanniemi SM, Levoska S, et al. Long-term effectiveness of bone-setting, light exercise therapy, and physiotherapy for prolonged back pain: a randomized controlled trial. J Manipulative Physiol Ther 2002;25: 99–104.

54. Hondras MA, Long CR, Cao Y, et al. A randomized controlled trial comparing 2 types of spinal manipulation and minimal conservative medical care for adults 55 years and older with subacute or chronic low back pain. J Manipulative Physiol Ther 2009;32:330–43.

55. Hsieh CY, Adams AH, Tobis J, et al. Effectiveness of four conservative treatments for subacute low back pain: a randomized clinical trial. Spine 2002;27(11):1142–8.

56. Hurwitz EL, Morgenstern H, Harber P, et al. A randomized trial of medical care with and without physical therapy and chiropractic care with and without physical modalities for patients with low back pain: 6-month follow-up outcomes from the UCLA low back pain study. Spine 2002;27(20):2193–204.

57. Mohseni-Bandpei MA, Critchley J, Staunton T, et al. A prospective randomised controlled trial of spinal manipulation and ultrasound in the treatment of chronic low back pain. Physiotherapy 2006;92(1):34–42.

58. Paatelma M, Kilpilkoski S, Simonen R, et al. Orthopaedic manual therapy, McKenzie method or advice-only for low back pain in working adults: a randomized controlled trial with one-year follow-up. J Rehabil Med 2008;40:858–63.

59. Rasmussen-Barr E, Nilsson-Wikmar L, Arvidsson I. Stabilizing training compared with manual treatment in sub-acute and chronic low-back pain. Man Ther 2003; 8(4):233–41.

60. Skillgate E, Vingard E, Alfredsson L. Naprapathic manual therapy or evidence-based care for back and neck pain: a randomized, controlled trial. Clin J Pain 2007;23(5):431–9.

61. Wilkey A, Gregory M, Byfield D, et al. A comparison between chiropractic management and pain clinic management for chronic low-back pain in a national health service outpatient clinic. J Altern Complement Med 2008;14(5):465–73.

62. Zaproudina N, Hietikko T, Hanninen OO, et al. Effectiveness of traditional bone setting in treating chronic low back pain: a randomized pilot trial. Complement Ther Med 2009;17:23–8.

63. Rasmussen J, Laetgaard J, Lindecrona AL, et al. Manipulation does not add to the effect of extension exercises in chronic low-back pain (LBP). A randomized, controlled, double-blind study. Joint Bone Spine 2008;75(6):708–13.

64. Evans DP, Burke MS, Lloyd KN, et al. Lumbar spinal manipulation on trial. Part 1: clinical assessment. Rheumatol Rehabil 1978;17:46–53.
65. Alderman D. Prolotherapy. In: Weintraub MI, editor. Complementary and integrative medicine in pain management. New York: Springer; 2008. p. 386.
66. Banks AR. A rational for prolotherapy. Journal of Orthopaedic Medicine 1991; 13(3):54–9.
67. Klein RG, Eek BCJ. Prolotherapy: an alternative approach to managing low back pain. J Muscoskel Med 1997;14(5):45–59.
68. Dechow E, Davies RK, Carr AJ, et al. A randomized, double-blind, placebo-controlled trial of sclerosing injections in patients with chronic low back pain. Rheumatology 1999;38:1255–9.
69. Mathews JA, Mills SB, Jenkins VM, et al. Back pain and sciatica: controlled trials of manipulation, traction, sclerosant and epidural injections. Br J Rheumatol 1987;26(6):416–23.
70. Yelland MJ, Glasziou PP, Bogduk N, et al. Prolotherapy injections, saline injections and exercises for chronic low back pain: a randomised trial. Spine 2004; 29(1):9–16.
71. Klein RG, Eek BC, DeLong WB, et al. A randomized double-blind trial of dextrose-glycerine-phenol injections for chronic low back pain. J Spinal Disord 1993;6(1): 23–33.
72. Ongley MJ, Klein RG, Dorman TA, et al. A new approach to the management of low back pain. Lancet 1987;2(8551):143–6.
73. Kovacs FM, Llobera J, Abraira V, et al. Effectiveness and cost-effectiveness analysis of neuroreflexotherapy for subacute and chronic low back pain in routine general practice. Spine 2002;27(11):1149–59.
74. Urrutia G, Burton K, Morral A, et al. Neuroreflexotherapy for nonspecific low back pain. Spine 2005;30(6):E148–53.
75. Keitel W, Frerick H, Kun U, et al. Capsicum pain plaster in chronic nonspecific low back pain. Arzneimittelforschung 2001;51(11):896–903.
76. Chrubasik S, Zimpfer CH, Schutt U, et al. Effectiveness of *Harpagophytum procumbens* in the treatment of acute low back pain. Phytomedicine 1996;3:1–10.
77. Chrubasik S, Junck H, Breitschwerdt H, et al. Effectiveness of *Harpagophytum* extract WS 1531 in the treatment of exacerbation of low back pain: a randomized, placebo-controlled, double-blind study. Eur J Anaesthesiol 1999;16:118–29.
78. Chrubasik S, Model A, Black A, et al. A randomized double-blind pilot study comparing Doloteffin and Vioxx in the treatment of low back pain. Rheumatology 2003;42:141–8.
79. Chrubasik S, Eisenberg E, Balan E, et al. Treatment of low back pain exacerbations with willow bark extract: a randomized double-blind study. Am J Med 2000;109:9–14.
80. Krivoy N, Pavlotzky E, Chrubasik S, et al. Effects of salicis cortex extract on human platelet aggregation. Planta Med 2000;67:209–12.
81. Chrubasik S, Kunzel O, Model A, et al. Treatment of low back pain with a herbal or synthetic antirheumatic: a randomized controlled study. Willow bark extract for low back pain. Rheumatology 2001;40:1388–93.
82. Ginsberg F, Famaey JP. A double-blind study of topical massage with Rado-Salil ointment in mechanical low back pain. J Int Med Res 1987;15:148–53.
83. Frerick H, Keitel W, Kuhn U, et al. Topical treatment of chronic low back pain with a capsicum plaster. Pain 2003;106:59–64.
84. Stam C, Bonnet MS, van Haselen RA. The efficacy and safety of a homeopathic gel in the treatment of acute low back pain: a multi-centre, randomized, double-blind comparative clinical trial. Br Homeopath J 2001;90:21–8.

Working with Pain Clinics and Other Consultants Concerning Low Back Pain

José E. Rodríguez, MD

KEYWORDS

- Low back pain • Referrals • Pain clinics

KEY POINTS

- While there are many treatments for back pain, working with consultants for the benefit of the patient is essential for quality treatment. Cooperation with consultants on the identification of risk factors for aberrant behavior and substance abuse is an important patient safety issue, for which the treatment team can effectively prevent harm.
- Back schools, physical and occupational therapy, ergonomic interventions, and patient education can all play significant roles in the recovery of the patient with low back pain.
- It is important for primary care physicians to maintain an active role in caring for patients with chronic pain. A constant conversation with the consultants is imperative. The primary care provider may not want to manage chronic pain but if left to specialists alone, the role of the primary care physician as a cohesive guide and caretaker can be lost.
- Know your consultants, talk to them frequently, keep abreast of new techniques and treatment regimens they are using, and be an active participant. Interprofessional collaborative and integrated care is the most important aspect of the management of chronic low back pain.

WORKING WITH PAIN CLINICS

Back pain is a very common complaint, and can be costly in terms of therapy and time away from work.[1] Although primary care physicians are able to manage low back pain, often it is necessary to refer to other specialists. This article discusses referral to pain clinics and working with other therapies.

In many states, Florida being a prime example, pain management has undergone intense scrutiny. While it is common for primary care physicians to manage chronic pain, many have chosen to work with pain clinics to provide better service to their patients, to decrease the intense scrutiny, or because many physicians find treating

Department of Family Medicine and Rural Health, The Florida State University College of Medicine, 1115 West Call Street, Tallahassee, FL 32306-4300, USA
E-mail address: Jose.rodriguez@med.fsu.edu

Prim Care Clin Office Pract 39 (2012) 547–552
http://dx.doi.org/10.1016/j.pop.2012.06.009
primarycare.theclinics.com
0095-4543/12/$ – see front matter © 2012 Elsevier Inc. All rights reserved.

patients with chronic pain to be unrewarding. Pain clinics exist principally to control pain. Many have the added benefit of being run by specialty-trained physicians who are certified in pain management, and provide an interdisciplinary approach.[2] Pain clinics are set up with safeguards to minimize abuse, such as frequent, random drug testing and pain-management contracts. These safeguards can be set up in primary care,[3] but the evidence supporting this practice is weak in the primary care setting.[4] There are many states that require certification of completion of extra training in pain management and opioid use. Pain clinics, however, are not without disadvantages: they can be costly, and although they can identify drug addiction and diversion, they do not always have the ability to treat these problems. Finally, communication between pain clinics and the referring primary care physician is often incomplete and intermittent.

Partners in group practice should avoid situations whereby savvy patients can play one partner against another. For example, one partner never gives opioid medications and refers to a pain clinic, and the other partner always gives opioids. It makes it easier if there is an office policy so that there is consistency of treatment. Solo practitioners should try to follow a similar consistent policy.

Specialists in pain management are like any other specialist. When consulted, referring providers should expect reports from every visit to the pain-management provider. If pain-management providers notice other problems with patients' medical management, they should indicate recommendations in their correspondence. Primary care providers should also be informed of the pain-management agreement that their patients have signed to include the type of treatments and medications, the doses, the dosing schedule, and any requirements to use a certain pharmacy. Primary care physicians can therefore work with pain-management providers for the enforcement of these agreements. Because narcotic pain medications have high abuse potential[5] as well as significant street value, providers should alert each other to behaviors that put patients at risk. The American Academy of Family Physicians pain-management monograph has an excellent list of these behaviors (**Box 1**). If patients exhibit these behaviors, action is necessary to increase patient safety and reduce physician liability.[6]

As providers identify patients who exhibit these behaviors, it is important to ensure that the patients receive adequate and appropriate treatment for the problems listed in **Box 1**. As a last option, the pain clinic provider may need to be notified and a discharge from the pain clinic arranged. Doctor shopping and pain-clinic shopping is common in patients with chronic pain. A statewide and, eventually, national registry of opioid prescriptions will help curtail misuse and diversion.

Pain clinics can be a valuable management tool for patients with chronic back pain. Not only can opioid use be closely monitored, appropriately prescribed, and regulated, but the pain clinic can offer multiple interventions and treatments based on an interprofessional model. Close communication with referring primary care physicians can result in a collaborative integrated model for the management of chronic low back pain.

BACK SCHOOLS AND WORKPLACE ERGONOMIC INTERVENTIONS

Patients also can benefit from other therapies that are not necessarily dependent on narcotic medications. Among these are back schools, ergonomic interventions, and physical/occupational therapy.

Back schools are educational interventions whereby patients with back pain are seen in group visits, during which patients learn back anatomy and function, posture,

---

Box 1
Aberrant behaviors of patients taking chronic medications for pain

Illegal or Criminal Behavior

- Diversion (sale or provision of opioids to others)
- Prescription forgery
- Stealing or "borrowing" drugs from others

Behavior that Suggests Addiction

- Use of prescription medications in an unapproved or inappropriate manner (injecting oral formulations, and applying topical patches to oral/rectal mucosa)
- Obtaining opioids outside of medical settings
- Concurrent abuse of alcohol or illicit drugs
- Repeated requests for dose increases or early refills
- Multiple prescription "losses"
- Repeatedly seeking prescriptions from other clinicians or emergency rooms after warnings to desist
- Evidence of deterioration in the ability to function at work, in the family, or socially
- Repeated resistance to changes in therapy despite clear evidence of adverse effects
- Positive urine drug screen—other substance use

Dangerous Behavior

- Motor vehicle crash/arrest related to opioid, illicit drug, or alcohol effects
- Intentional overdose/suicide attempt
- Aggressive/threatening/belligerent behavior in the clinic

Aberrant Behavior that Requires Attention

- Aggressive complaining about needing more of the drug
- Drug hoarding during periods of reduced symptoms
- Requesting specific drugs
- Openly acquiring similar drugs from other medical sources
- Unsanctioned dose escalation or other noncompliance with therapy
- Unapproved use of the drug to treat another symptom
- Reporting psychic effects not intended by the clinician
- Resistance to a change in therapy associated with "tolerable" adverse effects, with expressions of anxiety related to the return of severe symptoms
- Missing appointment(s)
- Not following other components of the treatment plan (physical therapy, exercise, and so forth)[6]

Adapted from Bittner B, Tenzer P, Romito K. Using opioids in the management of chronic pain patients: challenges and future options. AAFP Monograph 2010.

---

and mechanical strain. Abdominal isometric exercises and other exercises may be taught as well. These interventions were originally developed in Sweden. Patients can be seen weekly for up to 20 weeks, but shorter educational interventions may have benefit.[7] These interventions have shown benefit for up to 36 months.[8]

A recent Cochrane review included 19 randomized controlled trials (RCTs) studies of back schools as an intervention for low back pain. There were 3584 patients included in the review. Of the 19 RCTs reviewed, only 6 were considered to be of high quality (level of evidence A). Because of the wide heterogeneity of the studies, meta-analysis was not possible. The investigators concluded that there was moderate evidence suggesting that back schools can reduce pain and improve function in the short and intermediate term when compared with exercises, manipulation, myofascial therapy, advice, or placebo for patients with chronic low back pain. It was also concluded that the current studies have limited clinical relevance (Strength of Recommendation [SOR] B, systematic review of heterogeneous RCTs).[9]

Ergonomic interventions can prevent back strain from repeated lifting,[10] but a recent systematic review found that exercise was more effective for prevention of injury.[11] Although this is intuitive, it bears repeating that it is the most effective intervention to prevent injury. Prevention of injury while seated is a complicated and individual process. To be properly seated, measurements of the elbow, thigh, calf, and resting eye level are required. Using such measurements, a chair with low back support, adjustable arm rests, and knee supports can provide posture correction and thus prevent injury. However, the benefits of ergonomic office chairs may be limited, as the posture correction can diminish over time.[12] Also, workers may find the ergonomic chairs to be uncomfortable, which could reduce their use.[13] Such chairs are widely available, but can be very costly (up to $1000). Expense has thus proved to be an obstacle to the adoption of ergonomic chars in the workplace.

The ergonomic interventions are designed by occupational therapy and implemented in the workplace, usually by the employer. In one study of 825 nurses, an ergonomic workplace intervention was implemented to prevent injuries. The investigators provided a cost analysis and determined that it took about 3.75 years to recuperate the cost of the intervention and its implementation, in terms of the specialized equipment purchased. However, the intervention did result in fewer injuries to employees and a produced savings of $200,000 per year in workpersons' compensation costs. The intervention also resulted in higher job-satisfaction scores among employees.[14]

PHYSICAL AND OCCUPATIONAL THERAPY

Physical and occupational therapy (PT/OT) should be supervised by a physical medicine and rehabilitation physician. When referring to PT/OT, the same courtesies apply and the primary care physicians should be informed of treatment plans and progress. Primary care physicians should know what exercises are assigned and how often the patient should do them, and this can be an excellent resource to the specialist in helping to reinforce the messages of the PT/OT. Many insurance companies cover PT/OT, so patients need only to be referred to get treatment from these specialists. Patients receive PT/OT in 3 phases: acute, recovery, and maintenance.

During the acute phase of treatment, close communication between primary care and PT/OT is essential. Patients who are in pain are not likely to do the necessary exercises, so the primary care physician should provide pain control, or the patient should be receiving pain management from a specialist. Ideally this service would be offered on site, but in most instances the patient will travel to another site. Besides medical management PT/OT may use ultrasound, electrical stimulation, or specialized injections to treat the pain.

An expert panel from the American College of Physicians and the American Pain Society charged with composing treatment guidelines conducted a systematic review of nonpharmacologic treatments for pain. After analysis of 1292 abstracts, the investigators found 40 systematic reviews that met their inclusion criteria. Therapies reviewed included spinal manipulation, massage, acupuncture, exercise therapy, yoga, back schools, psychological therapies, multidisciplinary therapies, functional restoration, interferential therapy, low-level laser therapies, lumbar supports, short-wave diathermy, superficial heat, traction, transcutaneous electrical nerve stimulation, and ultrasound. The researchers found that only cognitive-behavioral therapy, exercise, spinal manipulation, and interdisciplinary rehabilitation showed any benefit for chronic or subacute back pain. Moreover, superficial heat therapy was the only treatment that produced benefit for acute back pain (SOR A, based on a systematic review).[15]

The recovery phase requires more specialized exercises. The object of the recovery phase is to restore full functionality. The process entails strengthening primary muscles, as well as strengthening accessory muscles to prevent further injury. During this phase patients typically need to learn new movements and different techniques to accomplish common tasks.

The longest and most difficult phase of PT/OT is the maintenance phase. During this phase the patient has full control, and success is dependent on the patient's commitment to the skills learned in the first 2 phases. For most patients, this also requires a commitment to physical fitness. Daily exercise, sensible sustainable dietary changes, and lifestyle modification are all parts of this phase. Stopping treatment during this phase is frequent, even though this is the most important part of treatment. During this time contact with the patient rests solely on the primary care physician.

While there are many treatments for back pain, working with consultants for the benefit of the patient is essential for quality treatment. Cooperation with consultants on the identification of risk factors for aberrant behavior and substance abuse is an important patient safety issue, for which the treatment team can effectively prevent harm. Back schools, PT/OT, ergonomic interventions, and patient education can all play significant roles in the recovery of the patient with low back pain. Managing patients with chronic low back pain can often be time consuming. There is also considerable risk for maladaptive behavior, psychosocial concerns, and aberrant or drug-seeking behavior. In addition, depression and anxiety are common comorbid diseases. It is important for primary care physicians to maintain an active role in caring for patients with chronic pain. A constant conversation with the consultants is imperative. The primary care provider may not want to manage chronic pain but if this is left to specialists alone, the role of the primary care physician as a cohesive guide and caretaker can be lost. Knowing consultants, talking to them frequently, keeping abreast of new techniques and treatment regimens they are using, and being an active participant are imperatives. Interprofessional collaborative and integrated care is the most important aspect of the management of chronic low back pain.

REFERENCES

1. Ivanova JI, Birnbaum HG, Schiller M, et al. Real-world practice patterns, healthcare utilization, and costs in patients with low back pain: the long road to guideline-concordant care. Spine J 2011;11(7):622–32.
2. Chen L, Houghton M, Seefeld L, et al. Opioid therapy for chronic pain: physicians' attitude and current practice patterns. J Opioid Manag 2011;7(4):267–76.
3. McCarberg BH. Pain management in primary care: strategies to mitigate opioid misuse, abuse, and diversion. Postgrad Med 2011;123(2):119–30.
4. Starrels JL, Becker WC, Alford DP, et al. Systematic review: treatment agreements and urine drug testing to reduce opioid misuse in patients with chronic pain. Ann Intern Med 2010;152(11):712–20.

5. Brown J, Setnik B, Lee K, et al. Assessment, stratification, and monitoring of the risk for prescription opioid misuse and abuse in the primary care setting. J Opioid Manag 2011;7(6):467–83.

6. Bittner B, Tenzer P, Romito K. Using opioids in the management of chronic pain patients: challenges and future options. AAFP Monograph 2010. p. 7.

7. Brox JI, Storheim K, Grotle M, et al. Systematic review of back schools, brief education, and fear-avoidance training for chronic low back pain. Spine J 2008;8(6):948–58.

8. Glomsrod B, Lonn JH, Soukup MG, et al. "Active back school", prophylactic management for low back pain: three-year follow-up of a randomized, controlled trial. J Rehabil Med 2001;33(1):26–30.

9. Heymans MW, van Tulder MW, Esmail R, et al. Back schools for non-specific low-back pain. Cochrane Database Syst Rev 2004;(4):CD000261.

10. Koltan A. An ergonomics approach model to prevention of occupational musculoskeletal injuries. Int J Occup Saf Ergon 2009;15(1):113–24.

11. Bigos SJ, Holland J, Holland C, et al. High-quality controlled trials on preventing episodes of back problems: systematic literature review in working-age adults. Spine J 2009;9(2):147–68.

12. Goossens RH, Netten MP, Van der Doelen B. An office chair to influence the sitting behavior of office workers. Work 2012;41(0):2086–8.

13. Mueller GF, Hassenzahl M. Sitting comfort of ergonomic office chairs—developed versus intuitive evaluation. Int J Occup Saf Ergon 2010;16(3):369–74.

14. Nelson A, Matz M, Chen F, et al. Development and evaluation of a multifaceted ergonomics program to prevent injuries associated with patient handling tasks. Int J Nurs Stud 2006;43(6):717–33.

15. Chou R, Huffman LH. Nonpharmacologic therapies for acute and chronic low back pain: a review of the evidence for an American Pain Society/American College of Physicians clinical practice guideline. Ann Intern Med 2007;147(7):492–504.

The Disability Evaluation and Low Back Pain

Stephen Quintero, MD[a],*, Eron G. Manusov, MD[b]

KEYWORDS

- Disability • Social Security Administration • Low back pain

KEY POINTS

- Although disability and impairment determinations can be time consuming and emotionally draining for physicians, this service to patients and society can greatly improve quality of life.
- A thorough knowledge of the anatomy, physiology, psychology, and function of the low back is the foundation for the diagnosis and determination of impairment.
- Use of a standardized method to collect and evaluate data combined with thoughtful review of evidence-based information can assist the primary care physician in the process of disability determination in patients with low back pain.

As described in articles elsewhere in this issue by Manusov, the incidence and prevalence of low back pain is high, yet exact numbers are difficult to determine.[1] It is estimated that almost 11 million persons are unable to work in the United States and an additional 8.1 million persons are unable to work to their full capacity.[1] In an analysis of patient visits to family physicians in the United States from 1995 to 1998 in the National Ambulatory Medical Care Survey, back pain is the 13th most common diagnosis made during family physician visits. A diagnosis of back pain is coded in 2.7% of visits, and back pain is the leading cause of disability in the United States for persons younger than 45 years.[2–4]

Impairment is defined as a marked loss or change in an anatomic structure of the body, psychological function, or physiologic function, and can be temporary or permanent. Impairment can progressively worsen, improve or remain static, be intermittent or continuous, or vary in intensity. Disability is defined as how the impairment affects the ability of a person to meet the demands of life.[1] As defined by the Social Security Administration (SSA), under federal law tasked to administer the Social Security Disability Insurance (SSDI) program and the Supplemental Security Income (SSI) program, a person is disabled if the criteria listed in **Box 1** are met.

[a] College of Medicine, Florida State University, 1115 West Call Street, Tallahassee, FL 32306-4300, USA; [b] Southern Regional Area Health Education Center, C.E.A.S., 1601 Owen Drive, Fayetteville, NC 28304, USA
* Corresponding author.
E-mail address: Stephen.quintero@med.fsu.edu

Prim Care Clin Office Pract 39 (2012) 553–559
http://dx.doi.org/10.1016/j.pop.2012.06.011   **primarycare.theclinics.com**
0095-4543/12/$ – see front matter © 2012 Elsevier Inc. All rights reserved.

Box 1
Social security criteria defining disability

- The applicant cannot do work he or she was previously able to perform
- It is determined that the applicant cannot adjust to other work, because of medical condition(s)
- The disability has lasted or is expected to last for at least 1 year or to result in death

This is a strict definition of disability. Rules of the Social Security program assume that working families have access to other resources to provide support during periods of short-term disabilities, including workers' compensation, insurance, savings, and investments.

Available at: http://www.ssa.gov/dibplan/dqualify4.htm. Accessed November, 2011.

There are many organizations and third-party entities who are involved in determining disability such as the Veterans Administration, the US Government, businesses, health care providers, insurance carriers, attorneys, and workers. Because low back pain so commonly occurs, most primary care physicians will be involved in either caring for a patient with a disability stemming from low back pain, or determining the functional capacity or degree of impairment caused by low back pain. This evaluation includes determining when to return to work, or recommending compensation for low back pain. This article reviews the role of the physician in impairment and disability determination, offers an approach to evaluation, and provides a template for the physician's report of findings.

THE ROLE OF THE PRIMARY CARE PHYSICIAN

The primary care physician is often the medical evaluator of a patient with low back pain. The advantages of having a primary care physician act as an independent medical evaluator include obtaining a second opinion from a nonbiased physician, having a biopsychosocial approach to patients with low back pain, and allowing for a referral from a third-party source, such as an attorney.[1] Potential disadvantages of primary care physicians performing disability determination include less depth of knowledge in comparison with the specialist, a negative impact on the primary care model of the physician-patient bond, and the difficulty of primary care physicians in remaining neutral.

To maximize the advantages, primary care physicians have the required training in musculoskeletal medicine with a broad understanding of physiology, anatomy, and function as well as the effects of disability and pain on patients and their immediate surroundings. Evaluating physicians must determine the initiator of the evaluation request (judge, insurance, employer) and understand the nature of the request (diagnosis, prognosis, work capacity, residual functional capacity, or causality). The primary care physician must remain objective and render advice that is free of personal opinion or bias from a personal or professional relationship with the patient. The primary care physician can address the evaluation request in an objective manner based on a thorough patient history and physical examination.

The disability determination process can vary according to the third party involved in the process. Reasons to have a disability determination include human resources, employer, legal cases, workman's compensation, and insurance requests.[5] The disability determination process for Social Security, however, is the most common and can serve as a model. The whole process has become easier since access to electronic health care records have become more available. Social Security representatives may collect evidence by telephone, mail, or electronic health records. Essentially the application requires a description of the applicant's impairments, treatment sources, and other information associated with what is referred to as the "alleged disability." The patient should be asked the 5 questions listed in **Box 2**.

The process of disability determination for the SSA includes a review of evidence by the Disability Determination Services or by an administrative law judge in SSA's Office of Disability Adjudication and Review. It is noteworthy that there are other consultative examinations performed in addition to that of the physician. Psychologists, optometrists, podiatrists, and speech-language pathologists often render determination advice and provide contributing evidence.

Once all examinations are complete, an initial determination on whether an applicant is disabled under the law is rendered. The information is then provided to a physician for a consultative examination if necessary. After review of the medical information, if the applicant is found to be disabled, the SSA will compute the benefit amount and begins payments. If there is an unfavorable determination and the applicant is not found to be disabled under the rules of the law, the file is retained in case of an appeal. The applicant can appeal the determination through the Office of Disability Adjudication and Review (ODAR), where an administrative law judge makes the second appeal decision. The judge may require additional evidence from other sources, including another medical evaluation.

History and Physical Impairment Evaluation

The assessment of disability starts with a history, physical examination, and review of supporting evidence, on completion of which the physician will determine the severity of the condition, make an assessment of the impact of disease or loss of function, and how the loss affects functional ability. The history is often complex and rarely complete in the supporting documents presented by the patient. Disability often occurs over a long period of time, with multiple physician visits and diagnostic procedures, and complex interactions between cognitive, behavioral, and physical contributors. The physician must remain unbiased and rely on objective data, but conditions are often complex and laced with softer, subjective data. It is important to be aware of how many providers have seen the patient, the multiple procedures and medications the patient has tried, and how the impairment has affected his or her entire life. The key to disability determination with low back pain is to focus on current loss of function. The Department of Veterans Affairs, the SSA, and the Occupational Therapy Association are good resources for maintaining the focus by offering information and guidelines that focus on functional assessment.

Box 2
The 5 questions necessary to determine disability for the Social Security Administration application

1. Are you working?

2. Is your condition "severe"?

3. Is your condition found in the list of disabling conditions?

4. Can you do the work you did previously?

5. Can you do any other type of work?

In addition to the history of the injury, pain, past evaluations, and past treatments, the history should include associated signs and symptoms, including a description of the character, location, and radiation of pain, as well as any mechanical factors that incite and relieve the pain. The history should include prescribed treatments including name, dose, and frequency of any medications used, as well as the applicant's typical daily activities, symptoms of weakness, other motor loss, or any sensory abnormalities. Contributing mental illness, along with any use of drugs or alcohol that may have an impact on the condition, should be explored. A good understanding of past medical illness, past surgical illness, review of systems, activities of daily living, and activities independent of daily life is imperative.

The majority of the evaluation will include:

The applicant's general appearance, nutritional state, and any apparent skeletal or musculoskeletal abnormalities.

The orthopedic and neurologic findings. These should include:

a. A description of Muscle mass, mobility, strength, and deep tendon reflexes. Specific attention must be paid to the spine to include muscle spasms; limitation of movement of the spine, described quantitatively in degrees from the vertical position when there is significant limitation in motion; and straight leg raising, given quantitatively in degrees from the supine position and from the sitting position. Changes in sensation and deep tendon reflexes should be described regarding intensity and symmetry for tendon reflexes and 2-point discrimination, distribution of altered sensation, and vibratory and positional sensation changes.

b. If there is no abnormality of range of motion of any affected joint on gross examination, that fact, rather than the actual degree of motion, should be reported.

c. Strength should be quantified and the method described. The most widely used method involves recording from 0 to 5 as a fraction, with the numerator representing the applicant's performance and the denominator representing a normal performance (eg, 3/5).

d. The degree to which motor function is inhibited by spasticity, rigidity, or pain.

Muscle mass should be documented. When there is asymmetry, specific measurement must be reported. Atrophy must be reported in terms of circumferential measurements of both thighs and lower legs (or upper or lower arms) at a stated point above and below the knee (or elbow) in inches or centimeters. A specific description of atrophy of hand muscles may be given without measurements of atrophy, but should include measurements of grip strength.

Gait and station should be evaluated, including the applicant's ability to: tandem walk, walk on heels and toes, hop, bend, squat, arise from a squatting position, dress and undress, get up from a chair; get on the examining table; and cooperate during the examination. If radiographs or other laboratory tests are performed, the physician providing the formal interpretation as well as the results must be identified.

Rheumatologic disorders require a higher focus of attention. The spine examination must include: general observations of stance, gait, ability to dress and undress, climb on the examining table, grasp or shake hands; and ability to write. A careful joint examination should specifically include detailed notations as to the presence or absence of effusion, episodes of infection, periarticular swelling, tenderness, heat, redness, and thickening of the joints, the specific range of motion of the joints and back in degrees, as well as structural deformities. Specific range of motion of a joint and particularly the spine should be reported in degrees. If myalgias or other muscular complaints are present, an evaluation of the areas of muscle tenderness including tender points and trigger points should be documented.

The patient's level of education and a mental status examination should be documented. If mental allegations are included then the presence or absence of mental abnormality in terms of affect, concentration, and memory should be determined. Documentation can include signs of nervousness, personal hygiene, simple directions, and calculations.

Assessment of Impairment

Impairment assessment conclusions such as disability evaluation schedules for the low back are not evidence based and produce great inter- and intraexaminer differences.[6–8] The International Classification of Functioning, Disability and Health (ICF) is based on the biopsychosocial model of disease and corresponds to body functions and structures, activities and participation, and environmental factors. Although the ICF contains more than 1400 categories, there are core sets for low back pain. These categories are a result of international decision making and a consensus process based on evidence available. The ICF are comprehensive and include 798 categories that reflect the complex functional problems found in patients with low back pain. The core set is difficult to use because it is so comprehensive; however, limitations and restriction in activities and participation may be the most relevant to patients with low back pain and correspond to the domains of mobility and self care. The benefit of the ICF is that the health professional's perspective, the patient's perspective, the medical diagnosis, the intervention program goal, the long-term goal, body-structure function, activity, participation, and environmental and personal contextual factors all are considered in the impairment determination. Gone are the prior "negative" terms impairment, disability, and handicap. These terms are replaced by resource-oriented perspectives such as function, activity, and participation.[7]

Primary care physicians are often asked to render an opinion on functional capacity. If a patient has no job to which he or she may potentially return, the assessment and recommendations are general. Recommendations should describe no restrictions needed, a restriction to medium to light physical activity, sedentary activity only, or less than sedentary restrictions. If there is a job to which the patient can potentially return, the opinion with regard to functional capacity must address the physical requirements of that specific job. Often a physical therapist or occupational therapist must be consulted to evaluate the ergonometric and functional requirements of the job. Other than ICF there are no standardized methods or requirements of reporting functional capacity. **Box 3** outlines the basics of the recommendations.

Psychiatric assessment may be necessary either because there may be a comorbid disease with low back pain or because of the complex interaction of cognition, behavior, and function. Psychiatrists or psychologists are the preferred examiners for assessing impairment of mental health.[2] The challenge is evaluating possibly exaggerated or fabricated symptoms. Use of the ICF can facilitate this determination, as the set takes into consideration motivation, personal and environmental factors, participation, and long-term goals.[8] Formal neuropsychological assessment using standardized tests may provide supporting evidence for inadequate effort or exaggeration of cognitive deficits.

Primary Care Physician's Report

The disability evaluation report for patients with low back pain must be written with regard to the intended audience. A succinct and accurate description of the history and physical examination as described in this article will outline the problem, describe how the history and physical examination are related to the problem, provide an assessment of impairment and, finally, a functional assessment. Data provided should

---

Box 3
Basics for functional capacity recommendations

No restrictions: The gait is normal, the range of motion of the back is excellent, straight leg raise is negative, and the neurologic examination is normal. There are no restrictions in standing, walking, sitting, or bending, and the patient would be capable of lifting 50 lb (22.7 kg) occasionally and 20 lb (9 kg) frequently. There are no other postural or manipulative limitations.

Medium to light: The patient is limited to standing and walking 6 hours in an 8-hour work day with normal breaks. The gait is slow but within normal range. No assistive devices are necessary for ambulation. The patient would be able to sit for 6 hours in an 8-hour day with normal breaks. Lifting and carrying is limited to 10 lb (4.5 kg) frequently and 20 lb occasionally. The patient is able to kneel, crawl, or squat only occasionally. There are no other manipulative or environmental limitations.

Sedentary: The patient would be able to stand and walk for more than 2 hours and sit for 6 hours in an 8-hour day with regular breaks. The patient must use an assistive device for ambulation (cane). The patient can lift and carry items weighing more than 10 lb frequently. There are no other manipulative or environmental limitations.

Less than sedentary: The patient is restricted to standing and walking for less than 2 hours in an 8-hour day. There is decreased range of motion of the back and the patient can sit 6 hours in an 8-hour day. The wheelchair is medically necessary and muscle strength is decreased in bilateral extremities. The patient is limited to lifting 10 lb frequently and 10 lb occasionally. Postural limitations include bending, stooping, crouching, kneeling, and crawling, and these should be avoided altogether. Environmental limitations include driving because of the inability to sit, decreased range of motion, and muscle weakness.

---

be as comprehensive and specific as possible, including degrees of rotation, specific range of motion, areas of decreased sensation, measurements of atrophy, and quantification of strength. The impairment determination will be general in the absence of specific job requirements but should be specific as to limitations. The limitations should include a reason. For example, the patient can sit for 6 hours in an 8-hour day owing to limitations in the range of motion of the hip and marked decrease in strength of the upper extremities.

The report should answer specific questions raised by the third party. Causality in impairment is determined using legal terminology such as "more probable than not" or greater than 50% probability. It is difficult to determine exact future impairment, as improvement beyond expectations is common. However, it is possible to make a determination based on the bio-psychosocial model by considering all factors. Comorbid diseases, environmental factors, and family and social support structures frequently can greatly affect how much a disability can result in impairment. The primary care physician can use existing data, consultants, and knowledge of the multiple factors affecting patients to make an educated determination.

SUMMARY

Although disability and impairment determination can be time consuming and emotionally draining for physicians, this service to patients and society can greatly improve quality of life. A thorough knowledge of the anatomy, physiology, psychology, and function of the low back is the foundation for the diagnosis and determination of impairment. Use of a standardized method to collect and evaluate data combined with thoughtful review of evidence-based information can assist the primary care physician in the process of disability determination in patients with low back pain.

REFERENCES

1. Freburger JK, Holmes GM, Agans RP, et al. The rising prevalence of chronic low back pain. Arch Intern Med 2009;169(3):251–8.
2. Taiwo OA, Cantley L. Impairment and disability evaluation: the role of the family physician. Am Fam Physician 2008;77(12):1689–94.
3. Edwards RR, Doleys DM, Fillingim RM, et al. Ethnic differences in pain tolerance: clinical implications in a chronic pain population. Psychosom Med 2001;63: 316–23.
4. US Department of Health and Human Services. The Surgeon General's call to action to improve the health and wellness of persons with disabilities. Washington, DC: US Department of Health and Human Services, Office of the Surgeon General; 2005.
5. Disability evaluation under social security (Blue Book, September 2008). SSA Pub. No. 64-039; ICN 468600. September 2008.
6. Clark WL, Haldeman S, Morris JJ, et al. Back impairment and disability determination: another attempt at objective, reliable rating. Spine (Phila Pa 1976) 1988;13(3): 332–41.
7. Institute of Medicine. Workshop on disability in America: a new look. Washington, DC: National Academies Press; 2006.
8. Stier-Jarmer M, Cieza A, Borchers M, et al. How to apply the ICF and ICF core sets for low back pain. Clin J Pain 2009;25(1):29–38.

Pain Processing in the Human Nervous System

A Selective Review of Nociceptive and Biobehavioral Pathways

Eric L. Garland, PhD

KEYWORDS

- Pain • Nociception • Neurobiology • Autonomic • Cognitive • Affective

KEY POINTS

- Pain is a biopsychosocial experience that goes well beyond mere nociception. In this regard, identification of the physical pathology at the site of injury is necessary but not sufficient to explicate the complex process by which somatosensory information is transformed into the physiologic, cognitive, affective, and behavioral response labeled as pain.
- In the case of chronic low back pain, the magnitude of tissue damage may be out of proportion to the reported pain experience, there may be no remaining structural impairment, and physical signs that have a predominantly nonorganic basis are likely to be present.
- Pain, whether linked with injured tissue, inflammation, or functional impairment, is mediated by processing in the nervous system. In this sense, all pain is physical. Yet regardless of its source, pain may result in hypervigilance, threat appraisals, emotional reactions, and avoidant behavior. So in this sense, all pain is psychological.
- Our nomenclature and nosology struggle to categorize the pain experience, but in the brain, all such categories are moot. Pain is fundamentally and quintessentially a psychophysiological phenomenon.

INTRODUCTION

Pain is a complex, biopsychosocial phenomenon that arises from the interaction of multiple neuroanatomic and neurochemical systems with several cognitive and affective processes. The International Association for the Study of Pain has offered the following definition: "Pain is an unpleasant sensory and emotional experience

The author was supported by grant DA032517 from the National Institute on Drug Abuse in the preparation of this article.

College of Social Work, Trinity Institute for the Addictions, Florida State University, 296 Champions Way, Tallahassee, FL 32306-2570, USA

E-mail address: egarland@fsu.edu

0095-4543/12/$ – see front matter © 2012 Elsevier Inc. All rights reserved.

associated with actual or potential tissue damage, or described in terms of such damage."[1(p210)] Thus, pain has sensory and affective components, as well as a cognitive component reflected in the anticipation of future harm. The purpose of this review is to integrate the literature on the neurobiological pathways within the central, autonomic, and peripheral nervous systems that mediate pain processing, and discuss how psychological factors interact with physiology to modulate the experience of pain.

FUNCTIONAL NEUROANATOMY AND NEUROCHEMISTRY OF PAIN
Pain Processing in the Nervous System

When noxious stimuli impinge on the body from external or internal sources, information regarding the damaging impact of these stimuli on bodily tissues is transduced through neural pathways and transmitted through the peripheral nervous system to the central and autonomic nervous systems. This form of information processing is known as nociception. Nociception is the process by which information about actual tissue damage (or the potential for such damage, should the noxious stimulus continue to be applied) is relayed to the brain. Nociception is mediated by specialized receptors known as nociceptors that are attached to thin myelinated Aδ and unmyelinated C fibers, which terminate in the dorsal horn of the spine. Sufficiently intense mechanical stimulation (such as stretching, cutting, or pinching), intense warming of the skin, or exposure to noxious chemicals can activate nociceptors.[2] In turn, activation of nociceptors is modulated by inflammatory and biomolecular influences in the local extracellular environment.[3] Although under most circumstances transmission of nociceptive information results in pain perception, many physicians and patients are unaware that nociception is dissociable from the experience of pain. In other words, nociception can occur in the absence of awareness of pain, and pain can occur in the absence of measurably noxious stimuli. This phenomenon is observable in instances of massive trauma (such as that which might be incurred by a motor vehicle accident) when victims exhibit a stoic painless state despite severe injury, and conversely, when individuals with functional pain syndromes report considerable anguish despite having no observable tissue damage.

By contrast, perception of pain occurs when stimulation of nociceptors is intense enough to activate Aδ fibers, resulting in a subjective experience of a sharp, prickling pain.[4] As stimulus strength increases, C fibers are recruited, and the individual experiences an intense, burning pain that continues after the cessation of the stimulus. These types of experiences occur during the 2 phases of pain perception that occur following an acute injury.[2] The first phase, which is not particularly intense, comes immediately after the painful stimulus and is known as fast pain. The second phase, known as slow pain, is more unpleasant, less discretely localized, and occurs after a longer delay.

Activation of nociceptors is transduced along the axons of peripheral nerves, which terminate in the dorsal horn of the spine. There, messages are relayed up the spinal cord and through the spinothalamic tract to output on the thalamus. In turn, the thalamus serves as the major "relay station" for sensory information to the cerebral cortex.[5] Nociceptive pathways terminate in discrete subdivisions of thalamic nuclei known as the ventral posterior lateral nucleus and the ventromedial nucleus.[6] From these nuclei, nociceptive information is relayed to various cortical and subcortical regions, including the amygdala, hypothalamus, periaqueductal gray, basal ganglia, and regions of cerebral cortex. Most notably, the insula and anterior cingulate cortex are consistently activated when nociceptors are stimulated by noxious stimuli, and activation in these brain regions is associated with the subjective experience of pain.[7] In turn, these integrated thalamocortical and corticolimbic structures, which collectively have been termed the pain neuromatrix, process somatosensory input and output neural impulses that influence nociception and pain perception.[8]

Neurochemistry of Pain

Nociception is mediated by the function of numerous intracellular and extracellular molecular messengers involved in signal transduction in the peripheral and central nervous systems. All nociceptors, when activated by the requisite mechanical, thermal, or chemical stimulus, transmit information via the excitatory neurotransmitter glutamate.[9] In addition, inflammatory mediators are secreted at site of the original injury to stimulate nociceptor activation. This "inflammatory soup" comprises chemicals such as peptides (eg, bradykinin), neurotransmitters (eg, serotonin), lipids (eg, prostaglandins), and neurotrophins (eg, nerve growth factor). The presence of these molecules excites nociceptors or lowers their activation threshold, resulting in the transmission of afferent signals to the dorsal horn of the spinal cord as well as initiating neurogenic inflammation.[3] Neurogenic inflammation is the process by which active nociceptors release neurotransmitters such as substance P from the peripheral terminal to induce vasodilation, leak proteins and fluids into the extracellular space near the terminal end of the nociceptor, and stimulate immune cells that contribute to the inflammatory soup. As a result of these neurochemical changes in the local environment of nociceptors, the activation of Aδ and C fibers increases, and peripheral sensitization occurs.[10]

In turn, nociceptive signal transduction up the spinothalamic tract results in elevated release of norepinephrine from the locus coeruleus neurons projecting to thalamus, which in turn relays nociceptive information to somatosensory cortex, hypothalamus, and hippocampus.[11,12] As such, norepinephrine modulates the gain of nociceptive information as it is relayed for processing in other cortical and subcortical brain regions. Concomitantly, opioid receptors in the peripheral and central nervous systems (eg, those in neurons of the dorsal horn of the spine and the periaqueductal gray in the brain) result in inhibition of pain processing and analgesia when stimulated by opiates or endogenous opioids such as endorphin, enkephalin, or dynorphin.[13] The secretion of endogenous opioids is largely governed by the descending modulatory pain system.[14] The neurotransmitter γ-aminobutyric acid is also involved in the central modulation of pain processing, by augmenting descending inhibition of spinal nociceptive neurons.[15] A host of other neurochemicals is also involved in pain perception; the neurochemistry of nociception and central-peripheral pain modulation is extremely complex.

Descending Central Modulation of Pain

The brain does not passively receive pain information from the body, but instead actively regulates sensory transmission by exerting influences on the spinal dorsal horn via descending projections from the medulla.[16] In their seminal Gate Control theory of pain, Melzack and Wall[17] proposed that the substantia gelatinosa of the dorsal horn gates the perception of noxious stimuli by integrating upstream afferent signals from the peripheral nervous system with downstream modulation from the brain. Interneurons in the dorsal horn can inhibit and potentiate impulses ascending to higher brain centers, thus providing a site where the central nervous system controls impulse transmission into consciousness.

The descending pain modulatory system exerts influences on nociceptive input from the spinal cord. This network of cortical, subcortical, and brainstem structures includes prefrontal cortex, anterior cingulate cortex, insula, amygdala, hypothalamus, periaqueductal gray, rostral ventromedial medulla, and dorsolateral pons/tegmentum.[7] The coordinated activity of these brain structures modulates nociceptive signals via descending projections to the spinal dorsal horn. By virtue of the somatotopic organization of these descending connections, the central nervous system can selectively control signal transmission from specific parts of the body.

The descending pain modulatory system has both antinociceptive and pronociceptive effects. Classically, the descending pain modulatory system has been construed as the means by which the central nervous system inhibits nociceptive signals at the spinal outputs.[16] In a crucial early demonstration, Reynolds[18] observed that direct electrical stimulation of the periaqueductal gray could produce dramatic analgesic effects, as evidenced by the ability to undergo major surgery without pain. Yet, this brain system can also facilitate nociception. For instance, projections from the periaqueductal gray to the rostral ventromedial medulla have been shown to enhance spinal transmission of nociceptive information from peripheral nociceptors.[19]

Central modulation of pain may have been conserved across human evolution because of its potentially adaptive effects on survival. For instance, in situations of serious mortal threat (eg, in the face of war and civil accidents, or more primordially, when being attacked by a vicious animal), suppression of pain might enable a severely injured individual to continue intense physical activity such as fleeing from danger or fighting a deadly opponent. Yet the neurobiological linkages between the brain, the spinothalamic tract, the dorsal horn, and the peripheral nerves also provide a physiologic pathway by which negative emotions and stress can amplify and prolong pain, causing functional interference and considerable suffering.

COGNITIVE, AFFECTIVE, PSYCHOPHYSIOLOGICAL, AND BEHAVIORAL PROCESSES IN PAIN PERCEPTION AND REGULATION

In addition to the somatosensory elements of pain processing already described, cognitive and emotional factors are implicit within the definition of pain offered by the International Association for the Study of Pain. Pain perception involves several psychological processes, including attentional orienting to the painful sensation and its source, cognitive appraisal of the meaning of the sensation, and the subsequent emotional, psychophysiological, and behavioral reaction, which then feed back to influence pain perception (**Fig. 1**). Each of these processes are detailed here.

Attention to Pain

In the brain, attention allows salient subsets of data to gain preeminence in the competitive processing of neural networks at the expense of other subsets of data.[20] The goal-relevance of a stimulus guides attention to select and distinguish it from the environmental matrix in which it is embedded.[21] Thus, attended stimuli receive preferential information processing and are likely to govern behavior. In this sense, attention allows for the evaluation of salient stimuli, and facilitates execution of approach behaviors in response to appetitive stimuli or avoidance behaviors in response to aversive ones. Thus, depending on its salience to the survival of the organism, the object of attention elicits the motivation to approach or avoid while the resultant emotional state, as the manifestation of approach or avoidance motivations, tunes and directs attention.[22,23] By virtue of its significance for health and well-being, pain automatically and involuntarily attracts attention.[24,25] Yet pain experience varies according to the locus of attention; when attention is focused on pain, it is perceived as more intense,[26] whereas when attention is distracted from pain, it is perceived as less intense.[27]

Attentional modulation of pain experience correlates with changes in activation of the pain neuromatrix; for instance, attentional distraction reduces pain-related activations in somatosensory cortices, thalamus, and insula, among other brain regions.[7] Concomitantly, distraction results in strong brain activations in prefrontal cortex,

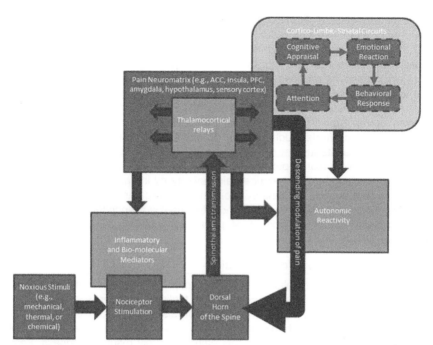

Fig. 1. Nociception, pain perception, and the biobehavioral response to pain in the human nervous system.

anterior cingulate cortex, and periaqueductal gray, suggesting an overlap and interaction between brain systems involved in attentional modulation of pain and the descending pain modulatory system.[28] By contrast, attentional hypervigilance for pain, a high degree of monitoring internal and external stimuli that is often observed among persons with chronic pain,[29] amplifies pain intensity and is associated with the interpretation of harmless sensations (such as moderate levels of pressure) as painfully unpleasant.[30,31]

Cognitive Appraisal of Pain

Pain involves a process of cognitive appraisal, whereby the individual consciously or unconsciously evaluates the meaning of sensory signals emanating from the body to determine the extent to which they signify the presence of an actual or potential harm. This evaluation is decidedly subjective. For instance, experienced weightlifters or runners typically construe the "burn" they feel in their muscles as pleasurable and indicative of increasing strength and endurance; by contrast, a novice might view the same sensation as signaling that damage had occurred. The inherent variability of cognitive appraisal of pain may stem from the neurobiological dissociation between the sensory and affective aspects of the pain experience; change in pain intensity results in altered activation of somatosensory cortex, whereas change in pain unpleasantness results in altered activation of the anterior cingulate cortex.[32,33] Thus, a sensory signal originating from the muscles of the lower back might be perceived as a warmth and tightness, or viewed as a terrible agony, despite the stimulus intensity being held constant. The manner in which the bodily sensation is appraised may in turn influence whether it is experienced as unpleasant pain or not.[34]

The extent to which a given bodily sensation is interpreted as threatening is in part dependent on whether the individual believes he or she is able to cope with that sensation. If, during this complex cognitive process of appraisal, available coping resources are deemed sufficient to deal with the sensation, pain can be perceived as controllable. Pain intensity is reduced when pain is perceived to be controllable, whether or not the individual acts to control the pain. Ventrolateral prefrontal cortex activation is positively associated with the extent to which pain is viewed as controllable and negatively correlated with subjective pain intensity. This brain region is implicated in emotion-regulation efforts, such as when threatening stimuli are reappraised to be benign.[35,36] Concomitantly, reinterpreting pain as a harmless sensation (eg, warmth or tightness) predicts higher perceived control over pain,[37] and psychological interventions have been shown to reduce pain severity by increasing reinterpretation of pain sensations as innocuous sensory information.[38] By contrast, pain catastrophizing (ie, viewing pain as overwhelming and uncontrollable) is associated with greater pain intensity irrespective of the extent of physical impairment,[39] and prospectively predicts the development of low back pain.[40]

Emotional and Psychophysiological Reactions to Pain

The aversive nature of pain elicits a powerful emotional reaction that feeds back to modulate pain perception. Pain often results in feelings of anger, sadness, and fear depending on the how the pain is cognitively appraised. For instance, the belief "It's not fair that I have to live with this pain" is likely to lead to anger, whereas the belief "My life is hopeless now that I have this pain" will likely result in sadness. Fear is a common reaction to pain when individuals interpret the sensations from the body as indicating the presence of serious threat.

These emotions are coupled with autonomic, endocrine, and immune responses, which may amplify pain through several psychophysiological pathways. For example, pain induction significantly elevates activity of the sympathetic nervous system, marked by increased anxiety, heart rate, and galvanic skin response.[41] Furthermore, negative emotions and stress increase contraction of muscle tissue; elevated electromyographic activity occurs in the muscles of the back and neck under conditions of stress, and negative affect and is perceived as painful spasms.[42,43] This sympathoexcitatory reaction coupled with emotions such as anger and fear may reflect an evolutionarily conserved, active coping response to escape the painful stimulus. Yet negative emotional states intensify pain intensity, pain unpleasantness, and pain-induced cardiovascular autonomic responses, while reducing the sense of perceived control over pain.[44] Stress and negative emotions such as anger and fear may temporarily dampen pain via norepinephrine release, but when the sympathetic "fight-or-flight" response is prolonged it can increase blood flow to the muscle and increase muscle tension, which may aggravate the original injury.[45] Alternatively, pain inputs from the viscera and muscles may stimulate cardiac vagal premotor neurons, leading to hypotension, bradycardia, and hyporeactivity to the environment, a pattern of autonomic response that corresponds with passive pain coping and depressed affect.[46] In addition to autonomic reactivity, proinflammatory cytokines and the stress hormone cortisol are released during the experience of negative emotion; these biomolecular factors enhance nociception, facilitate processing of aversive information in the brain and, when their release is chronic or recurrent, may cause or exacerbate tissue damage.[8,47,48]

Moreover, negative emotions are associated with increased activation in the amygdala, anterior cingulate cortex, and anterior insula. These brain structures not only mediate the processing of emotions, but are also important nodes of the pain neuromatrix that tune attention toward pain, intensify pain unpleasantness, and amplify interoception (the sense of the physical condition of the body).[49,50] Thus, when individuals experience negative emotions such as anger or fear as a result of pain or other emotionally salient stimuli, the heightened neural processing of threat in affective brain circuits primes the subsequent perception of pain[51,52] and increases the likelihood that sensations from within the body will be interpreted as painful.[53–55] The fear of pain, a clinical feature of patients with chronic pain, is associated with hypervigilance for and sustained attention to pain-related stimuli.[56] Thus negative emotions bias attention toward pain, which then increase its unpleasantness. In addition, negative emotions and stress impair prefrontal cortex function, which may reduce the ability to regulate pain using higher-order cognitive strategies such as reappraisal or viewing the pain as controllable and surmountable.[57,58] Thus anger, sadness, and fear may result from acute or chronic pain and in turn feed back into the biobehavioral processes that influence pain perception to exacerbate anguish and suffering.

Behavioral Reactions to Pain

Pain is not only a sensory, cognitive, and emotional experience but also involves behavioral reactions that may alleviate, exacerbate, or prolong pain experience. Typical pain behaviors in low back pain include grimacing, rubbing, bracing, guarded movement, and sighing.[59] These behaviors facilitate the communication of pain and exert social influences that may have vicarious gain for the individual suffering from pain; such benefits include sympathy, acts of kindness and generosity, tolerance, lowered expectations, and social bonding, among others.[60] In addition, guarding or avoidance of activities associated with pain may be negatively reinforcing by virtue of the temporary alleviation of pain experience.[61] The fact that these avoidant behaviors decrease the occurrence of pain results in increasing use of avoidance as a coping strategy. Yet, greater use of avoidance as a result of fear of pain predicts higher levels of functional disability.[62] It is not merely that persons with greater pain-related disability engage in more avoidant behaviors; rather, studies indicate that avoidant behavior and beliefs are a precursor to disability.[63–65] Avoidance contributes to negative clinical outcomes in patients with chronic low back pain. Fear-avoidance of pain influences physical impairment and is more strongly associated with functional disability than pain severity.[66–68] By contrast, progressive increase in activity through exercise has been shown to result in significant benefits in pain, disability, physical impairment, and psychological distress for patients with low back pain.[69] In light of the robust relation between coping behaviors and pain, behavioral and psychosocial interventions hold great promise in reducing pain intensity and pain-related functional disability in chronic pain conditions such as low back pain.[70]

SUMMARY

The foregoing review attests to the multidimensionality of pain. Pain is a biopsychosocial experience that goes well beyond mere nociception. In this regard, identification of the physical abnormality at the site of injury is necessary but not sufficient to explicate the complex process by which somatosensory information is transformed into the physiologic, cognitive, affective, and behavioral response labeled as pain. Indeed, in the case of chronic low back pain, the magnitude of tissue damage may be out of proportion to the reported pain experience, there may be no remaining structural impairment, and physical signs that have a predominantly nonorganic basis are likely to be present.[71,72] In this and other chronic conditions, to consider such pain as malingering or somatization would be to grossly oversimplify the matter. Pain, whether linked with injured tissue, inflammation, or functional impairment, is mediated by processing in the nervous system. In this sense, all pain is physical. Yet regardless of its source, pain may result in hypervigilance, threat appraisals, emotional reactions, and avoidant behavior. So in this sense, all pain is psychological. Our nomenclature and nosology struggle to categorize the pain experience, but in the brain all such categories are moot. Pain is fundamentally and quintessentially a psychophysiological phenomenon.

REFERENCES

1. Merskey H, Bogduk N. Classification of chronic pain, IASP Task Force on Taxonomy. Seattle (WA): IASP Press; 1994.
2. Brodal P. The central nervous system: structure and function. Oxford University Press; 2010.
3. Loeser JD, Melzack R. Pain: an overview. The Lancet 1999;353(9164):1607–9.
4. Bishop GH, Landau WM. Evidence for a double peripheral pathway for pain. Science 1958;128(3326):712–3.
5. Sherman SM, Guillery R. Functional organization of thalamocortical relays. J Neurophysiol 1996;76(3):1367.
6. Willis W, Westlund K. Neuroanatomy of the pain system and of the pathways that modulate pain. J Clin Neurophysiol 1997;14(1):2.
7. Tracey I, Mantyh PW. The cerebral signature for pain perception and its modulation. Neuron 2007;55(3):377–91.
8. Melzack R. From the gate to the neuromatrix. Pain 1999;82:S121–6.
9. Petrenko AB, Yamakura T, Baba H, et al. The role of N-methyl-D-aspartate (NMDA) receptors in pain: a review. Anesth Analg 2003;97(4):1108.
10. JM B. The neurobiology of pain. The Lancet 1999;353(9164):1610–5.
11. Yaksh TL. Pharmacology of spinal adrenergic systems which modulate spinal nociceptive processing. Pharmacol Biochem Behav 1985;22(5):845–58.
12. Voisin DL, Guy N, Chalus M, et al. Nociceptive stimulation activates locus coeruleus neurones projecting to the somatosensory thalamus in the rat. J Physiol 2005;566(3):929–37.
13. Yaksh TL. Opioid receptor systems and the endorphins: a review of their spinal organization. J Neurosurg 1987;67(2):157–76.
14. Basbaum AI, Fields HL. Endogenous pain control systems: brainstem spinal pathways and endorphin circuitry. Annu Rev Neurosci 1984;7(1):309–38.
15. Jasmin L, Rabkin SD, Granato A, et al. Analgesia and hyperalgesia from GABA-mediated modulation of the cerebral cortex. Nature 2003;424(6946):316–20.
16. Heinricher M, Tavares I, Leith J, et al. Descending control of nociception: specificity, recruitment and plasticity. Brain Res Rev 2009;60(1):214–25.
17. Melzack R, Wall PD. Pain mechanisms: a new theory. Science 1965;150(699):971–9.
18. Reynolds DV. Surgery in the rat during electrical analgesia induced by focal brain stimulation. Science 1969;164(3878):444.
19. Carlson JD, Maire JJ, Martenson ME, et al. Sensitization of pain-modulating neurons in the rostral ventromedial medulla after peripheral nerve injury. J Neurosci 2007;27(48):13222.
20. Desimone R, Duncan J. Neural mechanisms of selective visual attention. Annu Rev Neurosci 1995;18:193–222.
21. Corbetta M, Shulman GL. Control of goal-directed and stimulus-driven attention in the brain. Nat Rev Neurosci 2002;3:201–15.
22. Friedman RS, Förster J. Implicit affective cues and attentional tuning: an integrative review. Psychol Bull 2010;136(5):875.

23. Lang PJ, Bradley MM. Emotion and the motivational brain. Biol Psychol 2011;84: 437–50.
24. Legrain V, Perchet C, García-Larrea L. Involuntary orienting of attention to nociceptive events: neural and behavioral signatures. J Neurophysiol 2009;102(4): 2423.
25. Eccleston C, Crombez G. Pain demands attention: a cognitive-affective model of the interruptive function of pain. Psychol Bull 1999;125(3):356.
26. Quevedo AS, Coghill RC. Attentional modulation of spatial integration of pain: evidence for dynamic spatial tuning. J Neurosci 2007;27(43):11635–40.
27. Terkelsen AJ, Andersen OK, Mølgaard H. Mental stress inhibits pain perception and heart rate variability but not a nociceptive withdrawal reflex. Acta Physiol Scand 2004;180(4):405–14.
28. Wiech K, Ploner M, Tracey I. Neurocognitive aspects of pain perception. Trends in Cognitive Sciences 2008;12(8):306–13.
29. Schoth DE, Nunes VD, Liossi C. Attentional bias towards pain-related information in chronic pain; a meta-analysis of visual-probe investigations. Clin Psychol Rev 2012;32(1):13–25 [Epub 2011 Sep 17].
30. Hollins M, Harper D, Gallagher S, et al. Perceived intensity and unpleasantness of cutaneous and auditory stimuli: an evaluation of the generalized hypervigilance hypothesis. Pain 2009;141(3):215–21.
31. Rollman GB. Perspectives on hypervigilance. Pain 2009;141(3):183–4.
32. Rainville P, Carrier B, Hofbauer RK, et al. Dissociation of sensory and affective dimensions of pain using hypnotic modulation. Pain 1999;82:159–71.
33. Rainville P, Duncan GH, Price DD, et al. Pain affect encoded in human anterior cingulate but not somatosensory cortex. Science 1997;277:968–71.
34. Price DD. Central neural mechanisms that interrelate sensory and affective dimensions of pain. Mol Interv 2002;2(6):392–403.
35. Ochsner KN, Gross JJ. The cognitive control of emotion. Trends Cogn Sci 2005;9: 242–9.
36. Kalisch R. The functional neuroanatomy of reappraisal: time matters. Neurosci Biobehav Rev 2009;33:1215–26.
37. Haythornthwaite JA, Menefee LA, Heinberg LJ, et al. Pain coping strategies predict perceived control over pain. Pain 1998;77(1):33–9.
38. Garland EL, Gaylord SA, Palsson O, et al. Therapeutic mechanisms of a mindfulness-based treatment for IBS: effects on visceral sensitivity, catastrophizing, and affective processing of pain sensations. J Behav Med 2011;1–12.
39. Severeijns R, Vlaeyen JW, van den Hout MA, et al. Pain catastrophizing predicts pain intensity, disability, and psychological distress independent of the level of physical impairment. Clin J Pain 2001;17(2):165.
40. Picavet HS, Vlaeyen JW, Schouten JS. Pain catastrophizing and kinesiophobia: predictors of chronic low back pain. Am J Epidemiol 2002;156(11):1028–34.
41. Tousignant-Laflamme Y, Marchand S. Sex differences in cardiac and autonomic response to clinical and experimental pain in LBP patients. Eur J Pain 2006; 10(7):603–14.
42. Flor H, Turk DC, Birbaumer N. Assessment of stress-related psychophysiological reactions in chronic back pain patients. J Consult Clin Psychol 1985;53(3):354–64.
43. Lundberg U, Dohns IE, Melin B, et al. Psychophysiological stress responses, muscle tension, and neck and shoulder pain among supermarket cashiers. J Occup Health Psychol 1999;4(3):245–55.
44. Rainville P, Bao QV, Chrétien P. Pain-related emotions modulate experimental pain perception and autonomic responses. Pain 2005;118(3):306–18.

45. Cannon WB. Organization of physiological homeostasis. Physiol Rev 1929;9: 399–431.
46. Benarroch EE. Pain-autonomic interactions. Neurol Sci 2006;27(Suppl 2):s130–3.
47. Sommer C, Kress M. Recent findings on how proinflammatory cytokines cause pain: peripheral mechanisms in inflammatory and neuropathic hyperalgesia. Neurosci Lett 2004;361(1–3):184–7.
48. Chapman CR, Tuckett RP, Song CW. Pain and stress in a systems perspective: reciprocal neural, endocrine, and immune interactions. J Pain 2008;9(2): 122–45.
49. Craig AD. Interoception: the sense of the physiological condition of the body. Curr Opin Neurobiol 2003;13:500–5.
50. Wiech K, Tracey I. The influence of negative emotions on pain: behavioral effects and neural mechanisms. Neuroimage 2009;47:987–94.
51. de Wied M, Verbaten MN. Affective pictures processing, attention, and pain tolerance. Pain 2001;90(1–2):163–72.
52. Kirwilliam SS, Derbyshire SW. Increased bias to report heat or pain following emotional priming of pain-related fear. Pain 2008;137(1):60–5.
53. Bogaerts K, Janssens T, De Peuter S, et al. Negative affective pictures can elicit physical symptoms in high habitual symptom reporters. Psychol Health 2009; 25(6):685–98.
54. Panerai AE. Pain emotion and homeostasis. Neurol Sci 2011;32(Suppl 1):27–9.
55. Strigo IA, Simmons AN, Matthews SC, et al. Increased affective bias revealed using experimental graded heat stimuli in young depressed adults: evidence of "emotional allodynia." Psychosom Med 2008;70(3):338–44.
56. Keogh E, Ellery D, Hunt C, et al. Selective attentional bias for pain-related stimuli amongst pain fearful individuals. Pain 2001;91:91–100.
57. Arnsten AF. Stress signalling pathways that impair prefrontal cortex structure and function. Nat Rev Neurosci 2009;10(6):410–22.
58. Lawrence JM, Hoeft F, Sheau KE, et al. Strategy-dependent dissociation of the neural correlates involved in pain modulation. Anesthesiology 2011;115(4):844–51.
59. Keefe FJ, Wilkins RH, Cook WA. Direct observation of pain behavior in low back pain patients during physical examination. Pain 1984;20(1):59–68.
60. Hadjistavropoulos T, Craig KD, Fuchs-Lacelle SK. Social influences and the communication of pain. In: Hadjistavropoulos T, Craig KD, editors. Pain: Psychological perspectives. Mahwah (NJ): Lawrence Erlbaum Associates; 2004;87–112.
61. Turk DC, Flor H. Pain greater than pain behaviors: the utility and limitations of the pain behavior construct. Pain 1987;31(3):277–95.
62. Vlaeyen JW, Linton SJ. Fear-avoidance and its consequences in chronic musculoskeletal pain: a state of the art. Pain 2000;85(3):317–32.
63. Linton SJ, Buer N, Vlaeyen J, et al. Are fear-avoidance beliefs related to the inception of an episode of back pain? a prospective study. Psychol Health 2000;14(6):1051–9.
64. Buer N, Linton SJ. Fear-avoidance beliefs and catastrophizing: occurrence and risk factor in back pain and ADL in the general population. Pain 2002;99(3): 485–91.
65. Klenerman L, Slade P, Stanley I, et al. The prediction of chronicity in patients with an acute attack of low back pain in a general practice setting. Spine 1995;20(4): 478.
66. Crombez G, Vlaeyen JW, Heuts PH, et al. Pain-related fear is more disabling than pain itself: evidence on the role of pain-related fear in chronic back pain disability. Pain 1999;80(1–2):329–39.

67. Waddell G, Newton M, Henderson I, et al. A fear-avoidance beliefs questionnaire (FABQ) and the role of fear-avoidance beliefs in chronic low back pain and disability. Pain 1993;52(2):157–68.
68. Vlaeyen JW, Kole-Snijders AM, Boeren RG, et al. Fear of movement/(re)injury in chronic low back pain and its relation to behavioral performance. Pain 1995; 62(3):363–72.
69. Waddell G. Biopsychosocial analysis of low back pain. Baillieres Clin Rheumatol 1992;6(3):523.
70. Hoffman BM, Papas RK, Chatkoff DK, et al. Meta-analysis of psychological interventions for chronic low back pain. Health Psychol 2007;26(1):1.
71. Waddell G, McCulloch J, Kummel E, et al. Nonorganic physical signs in low-back pain. Spine 1980;5(2):117–25.
72. Waddell G. Low back pain: a twentieth century health care enigma. Spine 1996; 21(24):2820.

Medical-Legal Issues Regarding Patients with Low Back Pain

Shari Elizabeth Nokes*, Beau James Nokes

KEYWORDS

- Legal • Medical-legal • Low back pain

KEY POINTS

- Social Security Administration (SSA) defines disability as the inability to engage in any substantial gainful activity by reason of any medically determinable physical or mental impairment that can be expected to result in death or that has lasted, or can be expected to last, for a continuous period of not less than 12 months. Regarding lower back disabilities, a physician must usually be able to provide evidence that a low back problem meets the description of the medical impairment for SSA.
- Loss of function may be caused by bone or joint deformity or destruction from any cause; miscellaneous disorders of the spine with or without radiculopathy or other neurologic deficits; amputation; or fractures or soft tissue injuries, including burns, requiring prolonged periods of immobility or convalescence. The SSA Web site sets forth parameters for use when evaluating inflammatory arthritis or impairments with neurologic causes.
- Diagnosis and evaluation of musculoskeletal impairments should be supported, as applicable, by detailed descriptions of the joints, including ranges of motion, condition of the musculature (eg, weakness, atrophy), sensory or reflex changes, circulatory deficits, and laboratory findings, including findings on radiographs or other appropriate medically acceptable imaging. Medically acceptable imaging includes, but is not limited to, radiographs, computerized axial tomography, or magnetic resonance imaging, with or without contrast material, myelography, and radionuclear bone scans.

INTRODUCTION

Low back pain can present legal issues for a patient, and those legal issues frequently require input from and/or the participation of the patient's treating physicians. Because low back pain can lead to partial or complete disability, either on a short-term or long-term basis, patients can find themselves unable to earn a living the way they used to. This disability in turn may make it necessary for patients to seek benefits either in terms of government aid, personal insurance benefits, or insurance

This chapter is intended to provide general information concerning medical legal issues that commonly appear, but is not intended as a substitute for legal advice.

Nokes & Nokes, A Law Corporation, Main Office, 120 Vantis, Suite 520, Aliso Viejo, CA 92656, USA

* Corresponding author.

E-mail address: snokes@nokeslaw.com

Prim Care Clin Office Pract 39 (2012) 573–585

http://dx.doi.org/10.1016/j.pop.2012.06.012

primarycare.theclinics.com

0095-4543/12/$ – see front matter © 2012 Elsevier Inc. All rights reserved.

benefits through workers compensation or even, when the low back pain was caused by an incident that was the fault of a third party, through a personal injury claim lawsuit. Some benefits are based on the determination of how the disability affects the claimant's ability to work or find gainful employment. In addition to the financial consequences of disability such as lost earnings and medical bills, low back pain can greatly influence a patient's activities of daily living. A common element of tort damages that is sought by injury claimants is referred to as general damages. That term generally refers to the pain, suffering, emotional distress, humiliation, and embarrassment that can accompany a legitimate physical injury. In general, when an injured person makes a claim, the injured person's claim is not automatically accepted at face value by the person, company, or insurer against whom the patient makes a claim, and this is when a treating physician's input will be sought.

In many cases, a physician may even be hired to form an opinion concerning a client's injuries, medical care, and treatment. The hired expert scenario is beyond the scope of this article, but it bears mentioning because there may be an occasion on which a hired expert will review another physician's diagnoses, care, and treatment of a patient and will comment on whether or not that expert made appropriate diagnoses and provided proper care. In the experience of the authors, the physicians who provide the care and treatment of a patient are generally a better source of opinion concerning a patient's medical condition.

Most physicians do not go to medical school so that they can become involved in legal matters, but, because of the physician's vital role in diagnosing and treating low back pain, most physicians who address low back pain find themselves either asked to provide medical-legal opinions or compelled to discuss and justify their diagnoses by way of a subpoena.

Social Security Disability Claims

First, this article addresses social security disability claims, in which a patient is seeking benefits because of a disability that may or may not arise from a physical injury. The Social Security Administration (SSA) administers 2 programs that provide benefits based on disability: the Social Security Disability Insurance Program (title II of the Social Security Act [the Act]) and the Supplemental Security Income (SSI) program (title XVI of the Act).

Title II provides for payment of disability benefits to individuals who are insured under the Act by virtue of their contributions through the Social Security tax on their earnings, as well as to certain disabled dependents of insured individuals. Title XVI provides for SSI payments to individuals (including children less than 18 years old) who are disabled and have limited income and resources. SSA's criteria for deciding whether someone is disabled are not necessarily the same as the criteria applied in other government and private disability programs.

What is a Disability?

SSA's definition of disability is the inability to engage in any substantial gainful activity by reason of any medically determinable physical or mental impairment that can be expected to result in death or that has lasted or can be expected to last for a continuous period of not less than 12 months.

Regarding lower back disabilities, a physician must usually be able to provide evidence that a low back problem meets the description of the medical impairment for SSA. The government's Web site (http://www.ssa.gov/disability/professionals/bluebook) sets forth criteria for disability evaluation under Social Security (also known as the Blue Book) to provide physicians and other health professionals with an understanding of the disability programs administered by the SSA. It explains how each program works, and the kinds of information a health professional can furnish to help ensure sound and prompt decisions on disability claims. SSA also considers past work experience, severity of medical conditions, age, education, and work skills.

The following is a summary of the SSA guidelines, which are helpful when assessing patients with lower back conditions. The guidelines may change over time so it is a good idea to check the Web site for any changes.

Disorders of the musculoskeletal system may result from hereditary, congenital, or acquired pathologic processes. Impairments may result from infectious, inflammatory, or degenerative processes; traumatic or developmental events; or neoplastic, vascular, or toxic/metabolic diseases.

Loss of Function

Loss of function may be caused by bone or joint deformity or destruction from any cause; miscellaneous disorders of the spine with or without radiculopathy or other neurologic deficits; amputation; or fractures or soft tissue injuries, including burns, requiring prolonged periods of immobility or convalescence. The SSA Web site sets forth parameters for use when evaluating inflammatory arthritis or impairments with neurologic causes.

How loss of function is defined

Regardless of the cause(s) of a musculoskeletal impairment, functional loss for purposes of the listings is defined as the inability to ambulate effectively on a sustained basis for any reason, including pain associated with the underlying musculoskeletal impairment, or the inability to perform fine and gross movements effectively on a sustained basis for any reason, including pain associated with the underlying musculoskeletal impairment. The inability to ambulate effectively or the inability to perform fine and gross movements effectively must have lasted, or be expected to last, for at least 12 months. For the purposes of these criteria, consideration of the ability to perform these activities must be from a physical standpoint alone. When there is an inability to perform these activities because of a mental impairment, other criteria are to be used. SSA determines whether an individual can ambulate effectively or can perform fine and gross movements effectively based on the medical and other evidence in the case record, generally without developing additional evidence about the individual's ability to perform the specific activities.

What is meant by the inability to ambulate effectively?

Inability to ambulate effectively is defined as an extreme limitation of the ability to walk; that is, an impairment(s) that interferes seriously with the individual's ability to independently initiate, sustain, or complete activities. Ineffective ambulation is defined generally as having insufficient lower extremity functioning to permit independent ambulation without the use of a hand-held assistive device(s) that limits the functioning of both upper extremities. (An exception to this general definition may occur if an individual has the use of only 1 upper extremity because of amputation of a hand).

To ambulate effectively, individuals must be capable of sustaining a reasonable walking pace over a sufficient distance to be able to carry out activities of daily living. They must have the ability to travel without companion assistance to and from a place of employment or school. Therefore, examples of ineffective ambulation include, but are not limited to, the inability to walk without the use of a walker, 2 crutches, or 2 canes; the inability to walk a block at a reasonable pace on rough or uneven surfaces; the inability to use standard public transportation; the inability to carry out routine ambulatory activities, such as shopping and banking; and the inability to climb a few steps at a reasonable pace with the use of a single handrail. The ability to walk independently about one's home without the use of assistive devices does not, in itself, constitute effective ambulation.

What is meant by the inability to perform fine and gross movements effectively?

Inability to perform fine and gross movements effectively means an extreme loss of function of both upper extremities; that is, an impairment(s) that interferes seriously with the individual's ability to independently initiate, sustain, or complete activities. To use their upper extremities effectively, individuals must be capable of sustaining such functions as reaching, pushing, pulling, grasping, and fingering to be able to carry out activities of daily living. Therefore, examples of inability to perform fine and gross movements effectively include, but are not limited to, the inability to prepare a simple meal and feed oneself, the inability to take care of personal hygiene, the inability to sort and handle papers or files, and the inability to place files in a file cabinet at or above waist level.

Pain or other symptoms

Pain or other symptoms may be an important factor contributing to functional loss. In order for pain or other symptoms to be found to affect an individual's ability to perform basic work activities, medical signs or laboratory findings must show the existence of a medically determinable impairment(s) that could reasonably be expected to produce the pain or other symptoms. The musculoskeletal listings that include pain or other symptoms among their criteria also include criteria for limitations in functioning as a result of the listed impairment, including limitations caused by pain. It is, therefore, important to evaluate the intensity and persistence of such pain or other symptoms carefully to determine their impact on the individual's functioning. Descriptions and criteria for disability evaluation regarding the spine are listed in **Fig. 1**.

Disorders of the spine result in limitations because of distortion of the bony and ligamentous architecture of the spine and associated impingement on nerve roots

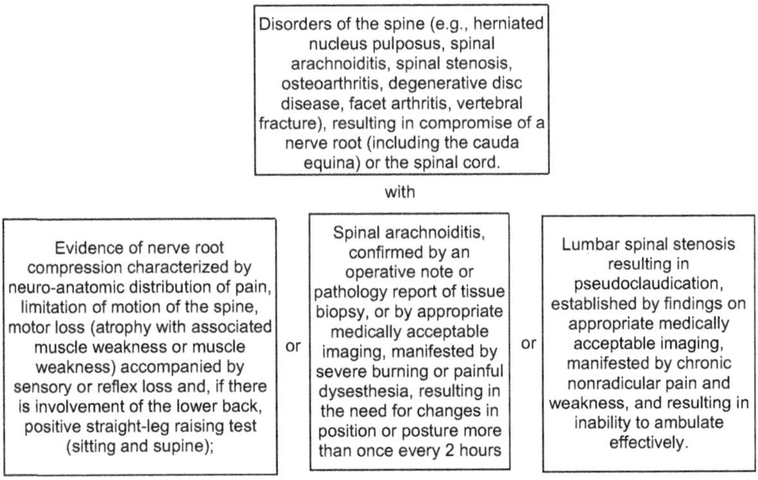

Fig. 1. Descriptions and criteria for disability evaluation regarding the spine.

(including the cauda equina) or spinal cord. Such impingement on nerve tissue may result from a herniated nucleus pulposus, spinal stenosis, arachnoiditis, or other miscellaneous conditions. Neurologic abnormalities resulting from these disorders are to be evaluated by referral to the neurologic listings in the SSA.

1. Herniated nucleus pulposus is a disorder frequently associated with the impingement of a nerve root. Nerve root compression results in a specific neuroanatomic distribution of symptoms and signs depending on the nerve root(s) compromised.
2. Spinal arachnoiditis.
    a. General. Spinal arachnoiditis is a condition characterized by adhesive thickening of the arachnoid, which may cause intermittent ill-defined burning pain and sensory dysesthesia, and may cause neurogenic bladder or bowel incontinence when the cauda equina is involved.
    b. Documentation. Although the cause of spinal arachnoiditis is not always clear, it may be associated with chronic compression or irritation of nerve roots (including the cauda equina) or the spinal cord. For example, there may be evidence of spinal stenosis, or a history of spinal trauma or meningitis. Diagnosis must be confirmed at the time of surgery by gross description, microscopic examination of biopsied tissue, or by findings on appropriate medically acceptable imaging. Arachnoiditis is sometimes used as a diagnosis when such a diagnosis is unsupported by clinical or laboratory findings. Therefore, care must be taken to ensure that the diagnosis is documented as described in 1.04B. Individuals with arachnoiditis, particularly when it involves the lumbosacral spine, are generally unable to sustain any given position or posture for more than a short period of time because of pain.
3. Lumbar spinal stenosis is a condition that may occur in association with degenerative processes, or as a result of a congenital anomaly or trauma, or in association with Paget disease of the bone. Lumbar stenosis is based on a decreased area that causes impingement on exiting nerves. Pseudoclaudication, which may result from lumbar spinal stenosis, is manifested as pain and weakness, and may impair ambulation. Symptoms are usually bilateral, in the low back, buttocks, or thighs, although some individuals may experience only leg pain and, in a few cases, the leg pain may be unilateral. The pain generally does not follow a particular neuroanatomic distribution; that is, it is different from the radicular type of pain seen with a herniated intervertebral disc, is often of a dull, aching quality, which may be described as discomfort or an unpleasant sensation, or may be of even greater severity, usually in the low back and radiating into the buttocks region bilaterally. The pain is provoked by extension of the spine, as in walking or standing, but is reduced by leaning forward. Patients with spinal stenosis often lean on a shopping cart or a walker, flexing at the waist to reduce the pressure caused by extension of the spine. The distance the individual has to walk before the pain begins may vary. Pseudoclaudication differs from peripheral vascular claudication in several ways. Pedal pulses and Doppler examinations are unaffected by pseudoclaudication. Leg pain resulting from peripheral vascular claudication involves the calves, and the leg pain in vascular claudication is ordinarily more severe than any back pain that may also be present. An individual with vascular claudication experiences pain after walking the same distance time after time, and the pain is relieved quickly when walking stops.
4. Other miscellaneous conditions that may cause weakness of the lower extremities, sensory changes, areflexia, trophic ulceration, and bladder or bowel incontinence include, but are not limited to, osteoarthritis, degenerative disc disease, facet

arthritis, and vertebral fracture. Disorders such as spinal dysrhaphism (eg, spina bifida), diastematomyelia, and tethered cord syndrome may also cause such abnormalities. In these cases, there may be gait difficulty and deformity of the lower extremities based on neurologic abnormalities, and the neurologic effects are to be evaluated under the criteria in the SSA.

Abnormal curvatures of the spine (specifically, scoliosis, kyphosis, and kyphoscoliosis) can result in impaired ambulation, but may also adversely affect functioning in body systems other than the musculoskeletal system. For example, an individual's ability to breathe may be affected, there may be cardiac difficulties (eg, impaired myocardial function), or there may be disfigurement resulting in withdrawal or isolation. When there is impaired ambulation, abnormal curvature of the spine resulting in symptoms related to fixation of the dorsolumbar or cervical spine, respiratory or cardiac involvement, or an associated mental disorder, there are other sections of the SSA that may be referenced. Other consequences should be evaluated according to the listing for the affected body system.

DIAGNOSIS AND EVALUATION CRITERIA

1. Diagnosis and evaluation of musculoskeletal impairments should be supported, as applicable, by detailed descriptions of the joints, including ranges of motion, condition of the musculature (eg, weakness, atrophy), sensory or reflex changes, circulatory deficits, and laboratory findings, including findings on radiographs or other appropriate medically acceptable imaging. Medically acceptable imaging includes, but is not limited to, radiographs, computerized axial tomography (computed tomography [CT] scan) or magnetic resonance imaging (MRI), with or without contrast material, myelography, and radionuclear bone scans. Appropriate means that the technique used is suitable to support the evaluation and diagnosis of the impairment.
2. Although any appropriate medically acceptable imaging is useful in establishing the diagnosis of musculoskeletal impairments, some tests, such as CT scans and MRI, are expensive, and attorneys do not routinely purchase them to support or refute their cases. Some, such as myelograms, are invasive and may involve significant risk. Attorneys do not request such tests as evidence. However, when the results of any of these tests are part of the existing evidence in the case record, they will consider them together with the other relevant evidence.
3. Consideration of electrodiagnostic procedures. Electrodiagnostic procedures may be useful in establishing the clinical diagnosis, but do not constitute alternative criteria to the requirements set forth earlier.

PHYSICAL EXAMINATION

The physical examination must include a detailed description of the rheumatologic, orthopedic, neurologic, and other findings appropriate to the specific impairment being evaluated. These physical findings must be determined from objective observation during the examination and not simply a report of the individual's allegation (eg, "He says his leg is weak and numb"). Alternative testing methods should be used to verify the abnormal findings (eg, a seated straight-leg raise test in addition to a supine straight-leg raise test). Because abnormal physical findings may be intermittent, their presence over a period of time must be established by a record of ongoing management and evaluation. Care must be taken to ascertain that the reported examination findings are consistent with the individual's daily activities.

Examination of the Spine

General

Examination of the spine should include a detailed description of gait, range of motion of the spine given quantitatively in degrees from the vertical position (0°) or, for straight-leg raise from the sitting and supine position (0°), any other appropriate tension signs, motor and sensory abnormalities, muscle spasm, when present, and deep tendon reflexes. Observations of the individual during the examination should be reported (eg, how an individual gets on and off the examination table). Inability to walk on the heels or toes, to squat, or to arise from a squatting position, when appropriate, may be considered evidence of significant motor loss. However, a report of atrophy is not acceptable as evidence of significant motor loss without circumferential measurements of both thighs and lower legs, or both upper and lower arms, as appropriate, at a stated point above and below the knee or elbow given in inches or centimeters. In addition, a report of atrophy should be accompanied by measurement of the strength of the muscle(s) in question, generally based on a grading system. A specific description of atrophy of hand muscles is acceptable without measurements of atrophy but should include measurements of grip and pinch strength.

When neurologic abnormalities persist

Neurologic abnormalities may not completely subside after treatment or with the passage of time. Therefore, residual neurologic abnormalities that persist after it has been determined clinically or by direct surgical or other observation that the ongoing or progressive condition is no longer present do not satisfy the required findings set forth earlier. More serious neurologic deficits (paraparesis, paraplegia) are to be evaluated under the criteria in the SSA.

DOCUMENTATION
General

Musculoskeletal impairments frequently improve with time or respond to treatment. Therefore, a longitudinal clinical record is generally important for the assessment of severity and expected duration of an impairment unless the claim can be decided favorably from the current evidence.

Documentation of Medically Prescribed Treatment and Response

Many individuals have received the benefit of medically prescribed treatment. Whenever evidence of such treatment is available, it must be considered. Some individuals not have received ongoing treatment or have an ongoing relationship with the medical community despite the existence of a severe impairment(s). In such cases, evaluation is be made from the current objective medical evidence and other available evidence, taking into consideration the individual's medical history, symptoms, and medical source opinions. Even though an individual who does not receive treatment may not be able to show an impairment that meets the criteria of one of the musculoskeletal listings, individuals may have impairments equivalent in severity to one of the listed impairments or be disabled based on consideration of their residual functional capacity (RFC) and age, education, and work experience.

These listings are examples of common musculoskeletal disorders that are severe enough to prevent a person from engaging in gainful activity. Therefore, in any case in which an individual has a medically determinable impairment that is not listed, an impairment that does not meet the requirements of a listing, or a combination of impairments no 1 of which meets the requirements of a listing, medical equivalence is considered. Individuals who have an impairment(s) with a level of severity that does not meet or equal the criteria of the musculoskeletal listings may or may not have the RFC that would enable them to engage in substantial gainful activity. Evaluation of the impairment(s) of these individuals should proceed through the final steps of the sequential evaluation process.

ORTHOTIC, PROSTHETIC, OR ASSISTIVE DEVICES
General

Consistent with clinical practice, individuals with musculoskeletal impairments may be examined with and without the use of any orthotic, prosthetic, or assistive devices as explained later.

Orthotic Devices

Examination should be with the orthotic device in place and should include an evaluation of the individual's maximum ability to function effectively with the orthosis. It is unnecessary to routinely evaluate the individual's ability to function without the orthosis in place. If the individual has difficulty with, or is unable to use, the orthotic device, the medical basis for the difficulty should be documented. In such cases, if the impairment involves a lower extremity or extremities, the examination should include information on the individual's ability to ambulate effectively without the device in place unless contraindicated by the medical judgment of a physician who has treated or examined the individual.

Prosthetic Devices

Examination should be made with the prosthetic device in place. In amputations involving a lower extremity or extremities, it is unnecessary to evaluate the individual's ability to walk without the prosthesis in place. However, the individual's medical ability to use a prosthesis to ambulate effectively, as defined earlier, should be evaluated. The condition of the stump should be evaluated without the prosthesis in place.

Hand-held Assistive Devices

When an individual with an impairment involving a lower extremity or extremities uses a hand-held assistive device, such as a cane, crutch, or walker, examination should be with and without the use of the assistive device unless contraindicated by the medical judgment of a physician who has treated or examined the individual. The individual's ability to ambulate with and without the device provides information as to whether, or the extent to which, the individual is able to ambulate without assistance. The medical basis for the use of any assistive device (eg, instability, weakness) should be documented. The requirement to use a hand-held assistive device may also affect the individual's functional capacity because 1 or both upper extremities are not available for such activities as lifting, carrying, pushing, and pulling.

When an individual is under continuing surgical management, this refers to surgical procedures and any other associated treatments related to the efforts directed toward the salvage or restoration of functional use of the affected part. It may include such factors as postsurgical procedures, surgical complications, infections, or other medical complications, related illnesses, or related treatments that delay the individual's attainment of maximum benefit from therapy.

EFFECTS OF OBESITY

Obesity is a medically determinable impairment that is often associated with disturbance of the musculoskeletal system, and disturbance of this system can be a major cause of disability in individuals with obesity. The combined effects of obesity with musculoskeletal impairments can be greater than the effects of each of the impairments considered separately. Therefore, when determining whether an individual with obesity has a listing-level impairment or combination of impairments, and when assessing a claim at other steps of the sequential evaluation process, including when assessing an individual's RFC, adjudicators must consider any additional and cumulative effects of obesity.

If a patient does not meet the definitions set forth earlier, the patient may prove disability based on limitations from any back disorder combined with any limitations from other conditions that prevent the patient from doing past relevant work. RFC Forms, also known as Ability To Do Work Related Activity Forms, may be used to show how the patient has limitations caused by a lower back condition in conjunction other medical conditions. If the patient cannot perform the duties of a previous occupation or a significant number of other jobs, SSA may find the patient disabled. GRID Rules set forth factors including age, education, and past work experience that are considered in determining disability. The GRIDs are a series of charts. The GRIDs consist of charts for sedentary, light, and medium levels of exertion. After SSA makes a finding on a patient's levels of exertion, SSA then looks at the corresponding chart and matches a patient's age, education, and past work and directs a finding of disabled or not disabled. SSA makes a determination as to the level of exertion at which a patient can perform in a work environment. The categories are from the lowest level of exertion to the greatest (ie, sedentary, light, medium, heavy, and very heavy).

If a patient is 50 years of age or older and past relevant work was performed at light, medium, or heavy levels and has no transferable skills, disability based on only back impairment is more likely. In this situation, the GRID Rules will direct a finding of disabled if the patient is limited to sedentary work. If the patient is younger than 50 years old, or 50 years or older and past relevant work is sedentary, the case is more difficult because the patient must show an inability to do sedentary work.

Inability to do sedentary jobs because of back disorders may be based on an inability to sit for more than short periods of time, inability to stoop, pain, or medication affecting the ability to concentrate or stay focused, and cervical radiculopathy affecting use of the arms or hands. It is also common for those with serious back impairments to suffer from depression.

BIOMECHANICAL/BIOMEDICAL ISSUES
Low Back Injuries from Low-Impact Automobile Accidents

Often a patient complains of lower back pain even though the patient may have been involved in a low-impact automobile accident. In legal cases, the likelihood of injury might be questioned because the lower back should be protected to a certain degree by the car seat. In these cases, the treating physician's opinion as to whether a particular complaint of pain is secondary to an injury caused in an automobile accident may be called into question. This challenge is frequently made by someone who does not have a medical degree and who relies on various statistical studies to state that a particular collision could not have caused a particular physical injury. Physicians who are busy treating patients are frequently unable to take the time to engage in lengthy study in biomechanics and so may think they are not qualified, or may feel insulted, when their diagnoses are called into question in a low-impact collision case. However, the physician's primary responsibility is to diagnose and treat the patient. In general, the opinion of a treating physician is going to be important to the patient. The issue of medical probability is addressed later in this article.

Malingering and Secondary Gain

Another issue that can arise is whether the patient is exaggerating the symptoms for gain, either financial or emotional. Attorneys or insurers defending against injury claims frequently raise secondary gain as an issue in cases involving claims of low back pain. This issue is best addressed by the treating physician, who knows the patient and who is familiar with the patient's history as well as the objective signs and symptoms shown by the patient.

Pain is subjective. This subjectivity is frequently pointed out when pain and injury become factual issues in a legal context. Treating physicians will probably be asked at some point whether they thought the patient had pain to the extent claimed. This situation is where personal observation and experience are valuable. There are tests for malingering, and those are generally done more frequently in a medical-legal context. The most prominent test is the use of Waddell signs.

There have been many articles written about Waddell signs and their usage, and this article is not a definitive reference on them, but does give a brief summary. Waddell signs are a group of physical signs, first described in 1980 in an article in *Spine*. Proponents of the use of Waddell signs think that the signs can indicate a nonorganic or psychological component to chronic low back pain. The signs have also been used to detect malingering. Testing takes less than 1 minute.

There are 5 categories of signs:

1. Tenderness tests: superficial and diffuse tenderness and/or nonanatomic tenderness
2. Simulation tests: these are based on movements that produce pain without causing that movement, such as axial loading and pain on simulated rotation
3. Distraction tests: positive tests are rechecked when the patient's attention is distracted, such as a straight-leg raise test
4. Regional disturbances: regional weakness or sensory changes that deviate from accepted neuroanatomy
5. Overreaction: subjective signs regarding the patient's demeanor and reaction to testing

When 3 or more categories contain a positive sign, the finding is considered clinically significant. However, use of Waddell signs has been criticized. For example, assessing the patient for overreaction raises the possibility of observer bias and discounts that each patient has idiosyncrasies, including reactions to pain.

Much has been written about Waddell signs, and the reader is encouraged to keep current on the medical literature surrounding this issue.

TESTIFYING IN PERSONAL INJURY DEPOSITION

Physicians will eventually be requested (or maybe even required) to give testimony concerning the care and treatment of their patients who have complained of low back pain. That testimony may be given at a trial or arbitration, or in a deposition.

What is a Deposition?

A deposition is the least cumbersome way to give testimony because it can usually be done at an office (particularly if you request that it be done there) instead of in court.

A deposition is a proceeding in which a physician testifies, under oath in front of a court reporter, responding to questions asked by attorneys. A deposition involves the same obligation to tell the truth as testifying in court in front of a judge and jury. In some circumstances, the deposition testimony can take the place of having to testify in person at trial. In other circumstances, expert witnesses hired by the parties can rely on a testimony in forming their opinions. And in any case in which a deposition is taken and a physician then has to testify at trial, anything said in the deposition can be read back in front of the judge and jury if the physician contradicts the earlier testimony. To avoid this embarrassment, physicians should stick to what they know (or have a good reason to contradict the deposition testimony, such as a later-discovered fact.) In general, physicians should give testimony that is precise, concise, and based on the care and treatment of the patient (as opposed to speculation).

Outside Research (Also Known as Homework)

Treating physicians are not required to do any research outside of their own care and treatment of their patients, so long as they have not agreed to act as hired expert witnesses in their patients' cases. This generally means that physicians do not have to form medical opinions other than those opinions formed as a part of the care and treatment of their patients. Those opinions may or may not be in their charts, but, if the opinion was important to the patient's care and treatment, they should be ready to explain why the opinions do not appear in the chart.

Do I Get Paid for this?

Many jurisdictions in the United States allow physicians to charge a reasonable hourly rate for the time they spend giving deposition testimony. Some physicians in jurisdictions that allow this have attempted to set an hourly rate so high that nobody wants to pay it, thereby hoping to avoid having to give deposition testimony at all. This practice has resulted in motions requiring doctors to come into court (or pay lawyers to go into court) to justify exorbitant hourly rates. The best practice is probably to become familiar with what other physicians in a given area of practice and geographic area charge. This preparation can save time and trouble (and can also help physicians make sure that they do not charge too little.) If a physician is an employee of a practice group, that group may already have set rates for testimony by its member physicians. In any case, physicians should tell the deposing party in advance what their hourly rate for deposition testimony is.

Can I/Should I Retain a Lawyer?

Deponents have a right to be represented by an attorney at deposition. In general, treating physicians who has done what they should have do not need one. However, many malpractice insurance carriers offer, at no additional charge, representation by counsel when called on to give a deposition. Physicians should at least check with their malpractice insurance carriers when they are asked to give a deposition.

Getting Ready for the Deposition

With a deposition, as with everything else, preparation is a good thing. Being ready for the deposition makes it go more quickly (so physicians can get back to taking care of patients) and will help ensure accurate testimony.

One thing you can do to speed the process is to keep your curriculum vitae (CV) current. Attorneys taking depositions always want details of the qualifications and experience of the testifying physician. The more cynical people who have been through this process tend to think that, because some attorneys bill by the hour, a painstaking and lengthy trip through their professional past is inevitable. However, a thorough and current CV can significantly shorten the deposition, particularly when the deposition is being taken by an experienced lawyer. The lawyer's chief concern is to make sure that the deposition contains enough information about a physician's professional background to qualify the testimony as admissible in court. When expert testimony is offered in court, a judge will not allow it into evidence until there has been enough information presented to show that the physician, as a doctor of medicine, is qualified to offer an expert opinion, such as a diagnosis or prognosis. If a current CV is offered when a physician is asked about qualifications and experience, many lawyers ask for confirmation that it is current and accurate, and then make it an exhibit to the deposition. This technique frequently shortens the deposition, although the lawyers may still want to discuss the aspects of a physician's professional experience that relate to the care and treatment of the patient.

Another thing that can make the deposition go more smoothly is to review the chart before testifying, including the records of other providers that were important in the diagnosis and treatment of the patient. The more a physician knows about a patient's history, the better (and as an added benefit this reflects positively on the physician as a health care provider.) The more the physician knows about the chart (and the better organized it is) the more quickly important entries can be found and the more quickly the deposition will be finished.

If a physician has agreed to be hired as an expert witness (this is usually to provide medical testimony for the patient and involves forming some opinions, based on medical literature or on records that did not need to be reviewed as a part of the care and treatment of the patient), there are usually additional requirements that must be met before the physician can give testimony, whether by deposition or in trial. These requirements vary depending on the jurisdiction in which the physician practices medicine, and the lawyer hiring/retaining the physician should know the specific requirements and help to provide the information necessary to meet them. As a general rule, if a physician keeps a log of information that will allow the disclosure of everything required by Rule 26 of the Federal Rules of Civil Procedure, there will be enough information on hand to make sure that the physician complies with the local rules of the jurisdiction.

TESTIFYING AT TRIAL

If you are called on to testify at trial, the same general guidelines concerning depositions apply. However, there are additional requirements that will apply if you have agreed to testify as a hired (retained) expert witness.

A patient's attorney might request that the physician act as an expert witness at trial. If physicians agree to act as an expert witnesses, they may have to do additional work to make sure that they will be allowed to testify. The attorney who wants to retain them should guide them through the process of providing the necessary information, but any physician should, as a matter of practice, keep certain things on hand (such as a current CV, as discussed earlier.) The Federal Rules Of Civil Procedure set forth requirements for expert witnesses who will testify at trial. When physicians are identified as retained expert witnesses, they must provide:

1. A complete statement of all opinions the witness will express and the basis and reasons for them
2. The data or other information considered by the witness in forming them
3. Any exhibits that will be used to summarize or support them

4. The witness's qualifications, including a list of all publications authored in the previous 10 years
5. A list of all other cases in which, during the previous 4 years, the witness testified as an expert at trial or by deposition
6. A statement of the compensation to be paid for the study and testimony in the case

In giving opinions, the physician may be asked to give an opinion, to a reasonable degree of medical certainty, regarding:

1. The nature of the problem, including diagnoses.
2. The cause of the lower back problem. For example, is the lower back pain caused by a degenerative condition, a sudden impact, or was a degenerative problem aggravated by an impact such as an automobile accident or work accident?
3. Whether the patient had an underlying condition that made him or her more susceptible to injury than a normally healthy person would be.
4. The prognosis for a full recovery from the lower back injury.
5. The nature and extent of any future disability the patient will have from any injury.
6. Future treatment, such as physical therapy, epidurals, or surgery.
7. The probability of success of the treatments.
8. The costs of necessary future treatments. The physician might be asked for an opinion regarding physician's fees, surgeon's fees, medications, hospital and anesthesia fees, and the like.
9. Whether medical treatment received was medically necessary.
10. Whether the charges for that treatment were reasonable for the local medical community.
11. To what extent the patient's medically necessary postaccident medical treatment was necessitated by injuries sustained in the event (such as an automobile accident), as opposed to any condition the patient had that predated the accident.
12. To what extent, if any, the patient's symptoms and medical treatment are attributable to aggravation of a preexisting medical condition. The physician will be asked to apportion how much of the patient's lower back problems are caused by a preexisting condition. If the patient did not need surgery before an incident, but did afterward, the physician might be requested to give an opinion as to whether the need for surgery is or is not the result of an accident.

The term reasonable degree of medical certainty is important. It can also be referred to as a reasonable degree of medical probability. It is usually considered the standard of proof in a civil lawsuit concerning a bodily injury. When a physician holds a medical opinion, the only way a judge or jury may be allowed to consider it is if the physician holds that opinion to a reasonable degree of medical certainty. The attorneys involved in the patient's case should be able to say what the standard of proof is in an injury case, but, in general, a reasonable degree of medical certainty translates to more likely than not, meaning that, the physician holds an opinion with a certainty of anything more than 50%; in plain English, if it is 50/50, that is not enough on either side (but, as a practical matter, whoever is suing has the burden of proof, meaning that the party has to prove the case by a margin of greater than 50%).

If asked to testify, the physician might consider having an outline or summary of opinions, with the basis for each opinion set out below each opinion.

Index

Note: Page numbers of article titles are in **boldface** type.

Prim Care Clin Office Pract 39 (2012) 587–593
http://dx.doi.org/10.1016/S0095-4543(12)00065-6
0095-4543/12/$ – see front matter © 2012 Elsevier Inc. All rights reserved.

primarycare.theclinics.com

Moving?

Make sure your subscription moves with you!

To notify us of your new address, find your **Clinics Account Number** (located on your mailing label above your name), and contact customer service at:

Email: journalscustomerservice-usa@elsevier.com

800-654-2452 (subscribers in the U.S. & Canada)
314-447-8871 (subscribers outside of the U.S. & Canada)

Fax number: 314-447-8029

Elsevier Health Sciences Division
Subscription Customer Service
3251 Riverport Lane
Maryland Heights, MO 63043

*To ensure uninterrupted delivery of your subscription, please notify us at least 4 weeks in advance of move.

Printed and bound by CPI Group (UK) Ltd, Croydon, CR0 4YY

03/10/2024

01040448-0012